On Being a Supervisee
Creating Learning Partnerships

Second Edition

Michael Carroll & Maria C. Gilbert

PSYCHOZ
PUBLICATIONS

First published in the UK 2011. This edition published in Australia 2011.

Copyright © 2011 by Michael Carroll & Maria Gilbert

PsychOz Publications
PO Box 124 Kew Victoria 3101 Australia
Ph: (61 3) 9855 2220 Fax: (61 3) 9855 2225
www.psychotherapy.com.au

Cover art by Savina Hopkins
Cover and text design by Cameron Crawford
www.cameroncrawford.com

National Library of Australia Cataloguing-in-Publication-entry:

Author:	Carroll, Michael
Title:	On being a supervisee: creating learning partnerships / written by Michael Carroll and Maria C. Gilbert
Edition:	3rd ed.
ISBN:	978 0 646 56335 0 (pbk.)
Notes:	Includes bibliographical references.
Subjects:	1. Human services personnel—Supervision of. 2. Human services personnel—Training of. 3. Medical personnel—Training of. 4. Interpersonal communication. 5. Learning.
Other authors:	Gilbert, Maria C.
Dewey Number:	361.007

PSYCHOZ
PUBLICATIONS

Contents

Preface to Second Edition

We are delighted our manual has survived and thrived through its birth, childhood and adolescence, and is now an adult. A second edition must be some sign of maturity. The first edition has sold out both here and in Australia where it was published separately. Developments in the world of supervision, education and neuroscience have added substantially to the literature and practice of supervision. We wanted to integrate up-to-date insights into the manual.

So, this is the turbo-charged version. We have updated it throughout and added two new sections. The first is a new supervisee skill: learning from experience. We now have seven supervisee skills. The second area of development is a larger and more elaborate section on reflection and, in particular, the six levels of reflection. In many ways these two sections have paralleled our own development where we are more aware than ever that supervision is about reflection on our experience and being facilitated to engage in reflective and collaborative dialogues on the experiences that arise from the work itself.

As ever, we continue to be educated by our supervisees, and enriched and fed by our annual BASPR (British Association for Supervision Practice and Research) conference. To our colleague Paul Hitchings (on the organising committee) we dedicate this second edition. He has been solid in friendship, unwavering in commitment and a wonderful and enjoyable colleague with whom to organise conferences. We would also like to remember Terri Spy who retired last year from the BASPR organising committee after many years of unstinting hard work. We wish her well in her post BASPR life.

It is often only in looking back that we all realise the joys of childhood and growing up. Being in the middle of it is hardly the time to appreciate it. It is true that 'youth is wasted on the young'. So with being supervisees. Sometimes it is in hindsight that we remember and enjoy the learning, struggling, experimenting and making mistakes of those early days. We believed we never could enjoy it while it was happening. Enjoy being a supervisee—it will soon pass. We hope this manual helps you in that enjoyment.

Michael Carroll & Maria Gilbert
June 2011

The Student's Prayer (Umberto Maturana)

Don't impose on me what you know,
I want to explore the unknown
and be the source of my own discoveries.
Let the known be my liberation, not my slavery.

The world of your truth can be my limitation,
your wisdom my negation.
Don't instruct me: let's walk together.
Let my richness begin where yours ends.

Show me that I can stand
on your shoulders.
Reveal yourself so that I can be
something different.

You believe that every human being
can love and create.
I understand, then, your fear
when I ask you to live according to your wisdom.

You will not know who I am
by listening to yourself.
Don't instruct me; let me be.
Your failure is that I be identical to you.

(Quoted in Zohar & Marshall, 2001)

Declaration of Supervisee Rights

As a supervisee, you have the right to:

1. Be respected for being a professional.
2. Become the professional you can be and want to be (and not a clone of your supervisor).
3. A safe, protected supervision space.
4. A healthy supervisory relationship.
5. Fair and honest evaluations and reports.
6. See your supervisor's reports on you with opportunity to comment on the contents.
7. Know what your supervisor thinks of your work.
8. Make good any areas of development outlined by your supervisor.
9. Clear and focused constructive feedback.
10. Give clear and focused feedback to your supervisor.
11. Ongoing, regular and systematic reviews of the supervisory arrangement.
12. Your own learning style.
13. Negotiate the supervision contract (and being aware, in advance, of what is not negotiable in the contract).
14. Mediation should the supervision relationship break down.
15. Appeal decisions made in supervision with which you have problems.

Declaration of Supervisee Responsibilities

As a supervisee you have responsibility for/to:

1. Your own learning.
2. Prepare for supervision.
3. Use supervision time effectively (manage time boundaries).
4. Present your work openly and honestly.
5. Deliver the best service possible to your clients or client group.
6. Create learning partnerships with your supervisor and other supervisees if there is a group.
7. Apply learning from your supervision to your work.
8. Be aware of other stakeholders in the supervisory arrangements, e.g., the families of clients, clients themselves, taxpayers, your profession, training courses, organisations (where applicable).
9. Monitor and evaluate your own work.
10. Reflect on your work.
11. Feedback to yourself and to others (other supervisees and the supervisor).
12. Be aware of cultural, religious, racial, age, disability, gender and sexual orientation differences between you and others.
13. Create ethical and professional environments for your work.
14. Where appropriate, give regular overviews of your work to your supervisor (the big picture).

Why this Manual?

'Though supervision is anticipated, there is little preparation for the experience' (Berger & Buchholz, 1992, p. 86).

'Despite both the overt and historical importance of supervision, new supervisees often have little formal preparation for the role' (Vespia, Hechman-Stone & Delwith, 2002).

There are lots of books on supervision, many of which support and help supervisors. There are almost none for supervisees, arguably the most important person in supervision. We will come back to that in a minute, but first, let us go directly to supervision.

The focus of supervision is learning. Supervisees learn from their work and from their supervision where they present their work in order that they may give a better quality of service to their client group. Supervisors are facilitators of learning. They aim to create the kind of collaborative relationship and the sort of learning environment that sustains learning for supervisees. Supervision is for supervisees, not for supervisors. Too often we have had to put up with supervisor-based supervision where supervisors take most of the initiatives, are motivated by their own current hobby horses, dazzle with their wisdom and insights, and take the spotlight off supervisees. This manual is to empower supervisees to take responsibility for their supervision and for their learning, and to persuade supervisors to allow them to do so.

This manual is primarily for supervisees. We consider a supervisee to be anyone, of any profession, who brings his/her work experience to another in order to learn from it. Supervisees come from professions such as psychology, social work, probation, nursing, psychotherapy and counselling (i.e., the helping professions) as well as from management, HR and Personnel departments. They may also be teachers, trainers, coaches, mentors, organisational consultants, tutors, spiritual directors and members of the emergency services or Prison Service. We are equally broad in seeing the focus of supervision as any aspect of the supervisee's work or professional development: direct coal-face contact (face-to-face contact) with individuals or groups; work with teams and organisations; programmes and training events; issues of continuing professional development; as well as relationship issues, process issues and even strategic elements of the work. We are aware of the many influences that impact on the actual work itself—all those can be valid focal points for supervision.

Most of the research in supervision involves supervisees. They have been asked, in all sorts of ways, what they think of supervision, what it means to them, how they view its various forms and expressions, how they see supervisors, and what are the features and characteristics of supervisors they find helpful and unhelpful. The number of questionnaires given to ascertain the views of supervisees is in stark contrast to the amount of help given them to use supervision effectively as a developmental tool. It is still rare for supervisees to receive help and instruction in being an effective supervisee. There is little literature to which supervisees can turn to help them to make sense of, understand and be, a collaborative partner in supervisory arrangements, either one-to-one or in a group/team. The best help for supervisees we have come across is the work of Inskipp and Proctor (2001) and Knapman and Morrison (1998), which brings supervisees systematically through what they need to know to use supervision effectively. However, the first work on supervisees (while being the most comprehensive and the classic in the field) is nested in Inskipp and Proctor's two working manuals on *'The Art and Craft of Supervision'* and, unless taken out and given to them by supervisors, would scarcely find its way into supervisee hands. Knapman and Morrison's self-development model for supervisees is a good initial start on the basics of being a supervisee—this manual builds on their work and asks supervisees to move further into understanding their own learning approaches.

Hence this manual. For supervisees (and for supervisors who want to know about being supervisees), it will lead you through the various stages of understanding, setting up, contracting for, maintaining and ending a supervisory relationship. The booklet agrees with the stances of Inskipp (1999) when she writes in her chapter on *'Training supervisees how to use supervision'*, that there are three reasons for concentrating on supervisees:

15. To empower supervisees.
16. To help supervisees be visible and transparent in supervision so that they are open and honest in what they bring (supervisors can only supervise what is brought to them).
17. To involve supervisees actively in all aspects of supervision so creating a collaborative learning relationship. To do this supervisees need skills, knowledge and practical ways to fulfil their roles and responsibilities (Inskipp, 1999).

Our hope is that this is a manual that supervisors and directors of training programmes will give supervisees for the above reasons and also because there is not enough time spent on helping supervisees use supervision effectively either on training courses or within supervision itself. However, while primarily for beginner supervisees (those who are still in training), this manual will also assist those who have been supervised before. Indeed, experienced supervisees might find it helpful to review how they take part in the supervisory relationship and the manual may help them look again at the various processes involved. It is too easy for all of us, no matter how experienced, to follow meaningless routines in our work no matter what our profession. This manual will provide a springboard for discussion—it cannot be an end in itself—between/amongst supervisees and supervisors so that they end up with the same understanding of supervision and are invested in the same supervisory outcomes.

Reading the manual

This manual is not intended to be read straight through from beginning to end. Different sections of it will be of help at different times in a supervisee's life. We have divided the manual into three sections to make it more accessible.

Section One is for beginning supervisees who may be thinking through supervision for the first time, and entering their first supervisory arrangements. It contains the basics of understanding supervision and being involved in choosing a supervisor (though some supervisees do not have that choice), as well as contracting and preparing for supervision.

Section Two contains material more applicable and useful to those who have begun supervision and have in place those elements discussed in Section One. From the strength of a healthy supervisory relationship, they can now look to other elements within supervision to enhance their learning of secondary skills (learning about developmental stages in supervision, what are 'drivers' and developing emotional literacy skills, amongst other themes).

Section Three is an Appendix which includes a number of exercises and frameworks to help supervisees as they move forward in supervision. Choose whichever suits you and makes sense for you at your stage of being a supervisee.

Our hope is that this manual will be a guide to you to make the best use of supervision. However, we are aware there are lots of areas within supervision that will not be covered, or if dealt with, will be done so in a short and concise way. Not because these areas are not important—some of them are essential to effective supervision—but because they may not be of direct immediate concern to you, the supervisee. Finally, we have no way of knowing what is and is not of interest to you in the area of supervision and do not want to confuse by being too 'all-inclusive'. So here are a few pointers to further information and reading if you find them interesting and helpful to your supervisory journey:

1. Is supervision effective? (Milne, 2009; Bambling, 2009).
2. Theories and models of supervision (Carroll, 1996).
3. Forms of supervision (Hawkins & Shohet, 2007).
4. Research in supervision (Ellis, 2010).
5. Setting up supervision (Inskipp & Proctor, 1993; 1995).
6. Group supervision (Proctor, 2008).
7. Supervision in context (Carroll & Tholstrup, 2001; Carroll & Holloway, 1999).
8. Training supervisors (Henderson, 2009).
9. Creative supervision (Lahad, 2000).
10. Developmental models of supervision (Stoltenberg & McNeill, 2010).
11. Pastoral supervision (Holton & Benefiel, 2010).
12. Supervision in organisational settings (Copeland, 2005).
13. Coaching supervision (Carroll, 2007; Hawkins & Smith, 2006).

We (the authors) are happy for you to contact us if there are other areas of supervision you would like to read up or know more about. See our biographies at the end for email contact.

While this manual hopes to 'empower' supervisees in all aspects of supervisory arrangements, we are all too aware that many supervisors and many organisations will not be supervisee-based. Quite the opposite, many supervisors will see no point in 'negotiating' with supervisees and will consider it their task to tell supervisees what supervision is and how they (supervisees) should involve themselves in it. Some hierarchical-based organisations will have little interest in setting up 'learning partnerships' but will work on the expert-beginner model of supervision, i.e., that it is the task of supervisors to tell supervisees how to do their work and guide and monitor that work, often concentrating on articulating weaknesses as a way to progress personal and professional development. We do not want to put supervisees in a 'no-win' situation, pretending that they will be partners in a learning endeavour when there is little chance of that happening. Having said that, we want to outline an understanding of supervision that, in our view, is based on solid principles of adult learning and will add value to both supervisees and their organisations while making supervision a much more interesting engagement for supervisors.

We repeat from earlier, supervision is for the learning of supervisees, and part of that learning is about *accountability*. Supervision is a process that accounts to whoever—clients, professions, authorities, managers, organisations, supervisors and supervisees—that supervisees take their work seriously enough to set up a reflective space within which they review their work, learn from it and apply that learning to their future work. Eventually supervisees will become reflective practitioners who reflect-in-action (think about the work as they do the work) and build on that reflection to do even better work.

Connor and Pokora (2007) have a chapter in their book on coaching on how to be an effective coachee (or client). We think their summary is worth remembering as a fine guide about what to keep in mind in order to get the best from your supervision and we have adapted their suggestions to the area of supervision.

1. Getting the right supervisor.
2. Knowing yourself.
3. Having realistic expectations.
4. Negotiating a working agreement.
5. Thinking ahead and being strategic.
6. Being proactive.
7. Learning from support and challenge.
8. Using reflective space.
9. Developing your imagination.
10. Identifying your resources and working smart.
11. Setting goals and making action plans.
12. Developing skills, making changes and delivering results.

(Connor & Pokora, 2007, p. 54).

CHAPTER 1

Overview of Supervision

What is a supervisee?

A supervisee is one who brings his/her work to another (individual or group) in order to learn how to do that work better.

Supervisees come to supervision:

1. for a variety of reasons (they have to or they want to);
2. choosing different types of supervision (peer, group, individual);
3. for various kinds of work (individual clients, groups, programmes, organisational) and;
4. with a raft of possible outcomes (accountability, reports, accreditation, training, consultation, better quality service for their client group).

Whatever the reason or the type of supervision, the actual work of the supervisee is at the heart of supervision. Supervision is about *'learning from doing'* or, *'becoming students of our own experience…sitting at the feet of our work'* (Zachary, 2002, p. xv).

Just in case you think supervision is only for helping professionals, have a look at the latest application of supervision. The American Military devised an interesting form of supervision they called the AAR (After Action Review). First tried in Kuwait and more recently in Iraq, it consists of commanders gathering their troops into small groups of 7–8 soldiers around them soon after military action has been completed. The commander first of all sets the ground rules, namely, that nothing any soldier says will be reported on his/her file and that no 'b' or 'f' words were acceptable (blame or fault). The commander then outlines six questions for open discussion:

1. What did we set out to do?
2. What happened?
3. What went well?
4. What went badly?
5. What have we learned?
6. What will we do differently next time?

Fifty percent of the time is spent on the first four questions and fifty percent on the final two with the commander taking notes of what was learned and what will be done differently next time. These notes are sent back to the CALL Centre (Centre for Army Lessons Learned) where they are collated and the new learning (information) is sent back to all units. The American Military has discovered the use of supervision under the title of 'The After Action Review'.

You are a supervisee. That means, in our view, that you have chosen to present your work to another (or others, as in a group) in order to learn from that presentation. There are a number of assumptions in the statement we have just made:

1. that you have 'chosen' supervision;
2. that you know how to present your work to another;
3. that you feel safe to present your work honestly and openly;
4. that you want to learn, and;
5. that you can trust your supervisor.

Exercise

You might want to think about some questions around those assumptions:

1. Is supervision something you 'have to do' rather than a process 'you have chosen to engage with'?
2. What has been your experience of supervision to date (as a supervisee), if you have already been in supervision?
3. If you have not been in supervision before, what immediately comes to your mind when you think of the term?
4. Do you have a clear understanding of what supervision means?
5. Have you considered how you learn and what learning style is best suited to you?
6. Has anyone ever talked to you, or have you thought about, how to present in supervision?

Let's look at some of your answers to these questions.

If your answer to the first question was that supervision is something you 'have to do', is mandatory because of your profession or the requirements of your work, and this is the only reason you involve yourself in it, PLEASE think again. Our experience is that doing something because you are required to do so rarely reaps as many benefits as it can. Sometimes quite the opposite—it blocks real learning and you will go through the procedure without heart or choice. Without apology we ask you to consider choosing to be in supervision, even if it is a requirement.

Choose supervision—it will make all the difference regarding your motivation and cooperation, and thus lead to more openness and learning. If you are or have been appointed a supervisor, and therefore have no choice as to whom he/she will be, you might like to look at helpful hints on how to handle this relationship on page 32.

If your experience of supervision has been *supervisor-centred* rather than *supervisee-based*, then we hope you might take a more *proactive* stance to negotiating what you want and need from supervision. Our hope is that the supervisor will move towards you, not insist that you move to join them in their way of learning and teaching.

We are also keen to help you *review your understanding* of supervision and what it has meant to you in the past.

And we will keep coming back to the focus of *learning* as the central aspect of supervision (not monitoring, or assessing, or evaluating, or giving feedback—all important dimensions of supervision, but not its key purpose).

Some of you reading this manual will be trainees in the process of learning your profession and who need the forum provided by an experienced person from the same profession to allow you to think through, reflect on and mull over the issues, problems and joys, that emerge from the work you are doing. Others of you will be qualified and experienced who, again, choose another person or group to be the recipient of your thoughts, ideas, and reflections on your work. In the conversation called 'supervision' you will look inwards to what is happening to you as you work and look outwards to how the work is being done. From these reflections will come learning that will be used to increase the effectiveness of the work.

While supervision has its roots in the helping professions, we consider that supervisees can come from any profession—what makes a supervisee a supervisee is a desire and wish to learn from opening up their work to others (whether it is as a manager, a Prison Officer or member of the emergency services, a spiritual director, a policeman or policewoman, a technician, a medical doctor, or even as a parent) so that in the ensuing conversation new thoughts, insights, awareness, ideas, feelings, approaches and theories will create better practice. Hence, we see the worlds of mentoring, coaching and consultation as closely allied to the world of supervision. We also see links here with line-management supervision. Even though roles and responsibilities can be different, the essence of all supervision is the same—how can I, as supervisor, facilitate the learning of supervisees from the actual work they do? From a supervisee's perspective the question is similar: How can I, as supervisee, present my work in the safe and facilitating environment of a healthy supervisory relationship so that I can learn from what I do?

What is supervision?

Our understanding is that you, as supervisees, come to supervision with a history of supervision—if not an actual experience of it then with some ideas or assumptions about it. You will have, already, an understanding or concept of what supervision should be or should not be—either from direct experience or from hearing others talk about it, or from the assumptions you make from hearing and using the term 'supervision'. It is important that you come to an agreed understanding with your supervisor about what supervision means.

Here are five definitions of supervision:

1. *'Supervision is a regular, protected time for facilitated, in-depth reflection on practice'* (Bond & Holland, 1998, p. 5).

2. *'Supervision is a working alliance between two professionals where supervisees offer an account of their work, reflect on it, receive feedback, and receive guidance if appropriate. The object of this alliance is to enable the worker to gain in ethical competency, confidence and creativity so as to give the best possible service to clients'* (Inskipp & Proctor, 2001).

3. *'Supervision is the construction of individualised learning plans for supervisees working with clients'* (McNulty, personal communication, 2003).

4. *'Supervision is a place of trust where a healthy relationship gives me a safe place to acknowledge and work with my work concerns, stresses, fears and joys'* (Johnson, personal communication, 2003).

5. *'When a person consults with a more 'seasoned' and experienced practitioner in the field in order to draw on their wisdom and expertise to enhance his/ her practice, then we would call this process supervision'* (Gilbert & Evans, 2000, p. 1).

When we take elements of these definitions together, supervision emerges with a number of features:

1. To ensure the welfare and best-quality-service for clients.

2. To enhance the personal and professional development of supervisees through ongoing reflexivity that results in advanced learning.

3. To gate-keep and monitor those who wish to enter and remain within their professions.

4. To benefit from the input of others as this applies to our work.

5. To draw on the wisdom and experience of another.

6. To build in accountability for the quality of the supervisee's work at all levels and to offer assurances to those who need to monitor that accountability.

Elements in supervision

A number of elements go to make up supervision. These include:

1. **A forum for reflection:** Supervision is the forum where workers reflect on their work and learn from that reflection through their interaction with another who takes on the role of supervisor. We will look in some detail later on what is reflection and how supervisors facilitate reflection.

2. **A forum for accountability:** Supervision is a process where clients' cases are presented and the supervisee's work with them is monitored, considered, reviewed, dissected with learning being brought forth. It also is a process of accountability where ethical and professional issues are considered and stakeholders in the supervision process (clients, organisations, professional associations and those who pay for the work) are assured that quality is being maintained.

3. **The focus is on experiential learning:** Experiential Learning is the type of learning most appropriate to supervision—not the only type, but the one used most often. Supervision is built on the reflection/action model where the practice of counselling/psychotherapy becomes the vehicle for learning. *The Experiential Learning Cycle* (Kolb, 1984) comprises four stages as shown in this diagram:

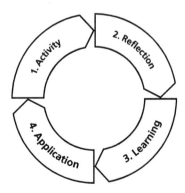

Figure 1: The Experiential Learning Cycle (Kolb, 1984)

1. Supervisees *do* their work—*'How are you doing your work?'* is the question asked by supervisors.

2. Supervisees *stop* doing their work and start *reflecting* on it—*'Are you able to reflect openly and honestly on your work?'* is the question to be asked at this stage.

3. Supervisees draw out their *learning* from their reflection—*What are you learning?*

4. Supervisees then *apply* their learning—*Do you implement your learning? Do you integrate this learning into your work activities?*

Supervisees can get stuck at any stage of this process—they may find themselves not able to engage in the activity, not able to reflect, not able to learn, not able to apply learning. The following are examples of individuals stuck at various stages of the Experiential Cycle.

Exercise

1. Jane is so stressed and overworked that she is unable to do her work as she would like. She is stuck at the *Activity Stage*.

2. Jack is so worried about getting it right, and being seen to get it right, that he cannot allow himself to consider areas of his work where he is not doing well. He is stuck at the *Reflection Stage*.

3. Jill gets stuck in the *Learning Stage* by not allowing herself to be vulnerable (and in a place of not knowing) so she cannot ask for what she needs in her learning.

4. Jim comes up with great ideas, but they never seem to get applied because he moves too fast and tries to do too much too quickly. He is stuck at the *Implementation Stage*.

Exercise

Consider the four stages of the *Experiential Learning Cycle* and where and how you sometimes get stuck. What do you experience when you get stuck? Is this a familiar place for you?

Experiential learning

The Experiential Learning Cycle (Kolb, 1984) has long been used as a framework for understanding how learning from experience takes place. Its four elements (*doing, reflecting, learning* and *applying learning*) work together to make learning from experience possible. The Experiential learning cycle integrates four ways of knowing:

1. **Tacit knowledge** (knowing intuitively) which is the foundation of 'doing' the work. In practicing our work we delve into the font of knowledge that we possess and intuitively, and hopefully from an 'unconscious competence' perspective, do our job well. Called in educational circles 'automaticity', intuitive knowing is the most effective way to engage in work. We know automatically and we practice intuitively. The difference between the amateur and the professional, or the beginner and the more experienced practitioner, is this intuitive ability. Beginners think about what they are doing, they watch themselves perform; they hover above themselves rationally deciding their next steps. Experienced practitioners tend not to do this, and instead dip unconsciously into their pool of tacit knowledge and intuitively know the best course of action. There is some evidence from sports coaching and sports psychology that the more we think about what we are doing when we are actually doing it, the more our performance deteriorates. The time for thinking and reflection is not during the process, but before and after the process has occurred. *'Just do it'* is a sensible injunction to those of us who over-reflect or monitor our actions as we do them. Schon (1983; 1987) calls this *'knowing-in-action'* or *'knowing-in-use'* (the ability to access our knowledge while behaving) and sees reflection-in-action as the process that allows us to do so.

2. **Reflective knowledge** (knowing why). Experiential learning involves using reflection as a method of learning. Reflection and critical reflective learning involves supervisees in honest consideration and investigation of their work (Mezirow & Associates, 2000). Supervisors facilitate this reflection by setting up an environment of inquiry in order to help supervisees learn from their own practice. With open mind and open heart (Scharmer, 2007), supervisees are transparent, honest, aware and alert to what is happening as they reflect on the procedures, processes and relationships involved.

3. **Propositional or declarative learning** (knowing that) now emerges from critical reflection. Learning is articulated and connected to theory, frameworks, models and other intellectual definitions and descriptions. Learning is captured in words and voices—articulating our learning in propositions and theories can focus our learning.

4. **Practical or procedural knowledge** (knowing how) emerges in the final section of the *Experiential Learning Cycle* in finding ways to translate propositional learning into skills, capabilities, competencies and qualities of the supervisee that enables him or her to return to the work. The application of knowledge is itself a form of knowing as we learn the practice skills of translating our theories into our work.

In their application of the *Experiential Learning Cycle* to coaching, Law, Ireland and Hussain (2007) outline three movements:

1. An internal to external movement—the internal movement involves reflection and conceptualisation of new learning. This, in turn, leads to the second external movement from action/application of learning to new practice.

2. A past, present and future movement—past experience is reflected on in the present which gives rise to new meaning that is then integrated into future work.

3. A 'movement within' which results in changing meaning—the meaning and interpretation of our experience changes as we hold it up to critical examination.

A further movement could be added—from *unconscious competence* (accessing our pool of tacit knowledge) through *conscious incompetence* (allowing ourselves vulnerability as we reflect on our work and translate that vulnerability into new learning) and into new applications of learning to our work (Clarkson & Gilbert, 1991). Moore (2008) focuses on the *emotional knowing* side of this work and presents a model where *'the reflexive, non-shaming learning environment of the process framework is at the service of facilitating firstly self-awareness through reflexivity, secondly other-awareness through empathy, and finally therapeutic awareness through reiterative empathy'* (p. 7).

Supervisors facilitate the learning of supervisees by ensuring that these blocks are dealt with and that learning continues around the *Experiential Learning Cycle*. A number of supervision features now emerge:

1. The focus of supervision is on the learning of supervisees, i.e., your learning. Hitherto the apprentice joined the master-practitioner, watched, learned, tried out the work, and was given feedback on how it should be done, practised and then learned more. Power, the right way to do the job and how this was taught, resided in the hands of the supervisor. The

new emphasis is on the learning of supervisees with supervisors interested in questions such as: At what stage in their professional development are supervisees? How do they best learn? What learning objectives supply the focus of supervision time? How are supervisees integrating the various components of their training and experience?

2. Your main learning takes place through reflection on the actual work itself.

3. Your supervisor is primarily a 'manager of learning' and hopefully asks questions such as: *"How can I, as supervisor, assist your learning?"*

4. Empowering you to be an active collaborator in the learning endeavour of supervision is essential for learning.

5. Supervision is an emotional experience as well as a rational one and the emotional aspect needs to be considered and worked with in supervision.

6. You will acquire your own style of being a practitioner. There is no objective way of helping (as there may be in becoming a carpenter, plumber or goldsmith, professions from which the apprenticeship models emerged). While there is a programme to be followed participants learn their way of doing it. Supervision is needed so that individuals can forge their own identity within the overall boundaries of the profession and the programme. Training is not about learning to do it as the supervisor does it, but about learning an individual and unique way of interacting with work.

7. You will go through stages on your journey to becoming an expert practitioner. Supervisors perform various tasks as they work with you. If these tasks can be geared to the developmental stage through which you are travelling then learning can be better managed and can be seen as cumulative.

Your own philosophy of supervision

At this stage, we hope you are ready to write your own 'philosophy of supervision', i.e., what it means to you. Can you capture in a paragraph what it might look like? One group of supervisees used images and metaphors to capture what supervision meant to them and came up with the following:

For me, supervision is:

1. A *'torch'*, which illuminates my work.

2. A *'container'*, where I feel safe and held.

3. A *'mirror'*, where I see myself and my work (the mirror is usually held by my supervisor).

4. A *'playpen'*, where we play with ideas, feelings, intuitions, hunches, theories.

5. A *'dance'*, where we learn how to work together in harmony.

6. A *'classroom'*, which contains two learners one of which facilitates my learning.

7. A *'courtroom'*, where assessments, evaluations and judgements take place.

8. A *'journey'*, where we both move through stages and need to decide where we are going, what we want to take with us, and what to leave behind.

9. A *'thermometer'*, to gauge temperatures (intellectual, emotional, psychological and social climates).

10. A *'sculpture'*, where I am being fashioned into something yet to be.

You might like to draw what supervision means to you. What images/symbols come to you when you think of what supervision might be? What is your image?

Exercise

In whatever way suits you, illustrate: *What supervision means to me is…* or you may prefer to answer the following series of questions.

Thinking through supervision

1. What has been my experience of supervision to date?

2. What do I want from supervision?

3. What do I want from my supervisor?

4. What learning objectives would I like to bring to supervision?

5. What worries me about supervision? My supervisor?

6. What are the kinds of problems that could arise within supervision?

7. What interests me about supervision?

Forms and contexts of supervision

So far, we have talked about supervision as if there was only one form of supervision. As you may know, there are a number of formats all of which have their strengths and limitations. While you may not have a choice about the kind of supervision in which you are involved, it is worthwhile reviewing the various forms. We want, briefly, to look at four:

8. **Individual supervision** (one supervisor and one supervisee). In this process the supervisee consults with one other person who is usually a more experienced member of the profession. One of the main advantages of individual supervision is that it provides you with the undivided attention of the supervisor. Some supervisees prefer this at stages of their development when they have particular challenges to face or when they get shamed easily in front of peers if there is any critical feedback to be given (See Carroll, 1996; Gilbert & Evans, 2000, for further reading on this area of supervision).

9. **Group supervision** (one supervisor and several supervisees). The advantage of this form of supervision is that the supervisee gets the benefit of feedback from peers as well as learning from the variety of work that is presented by others in the group. In our experience, many supervisees enjoy this form of supervision because of the variety of input and the additional sense of support that comes from belonging to a small community of peers (Proctor's 2008 book, *Group Supervision*, is the best for those wanting to know more about this form of supervision).

10. **Peer supervision** (two or more people in a group where there is no designated supervisor but each participant becomes co-supervisor and supervisee at different times). The advantage of this form of supervision is that it provides you with the opportunity to interact with people at your level of development and share one another's fears and triumphs. Many people combine this arrangement with individual or group supervision to gain extra support (see Hawkins & Shohet, 2000 for further insights into peer group supervision).

11. **Team supervision**—where the group, in this instance, is also a team that works together. The advantage of this form of supervision is that it provides the team with a safe place where issues can be brought and worked through in the presence of a facilitator, the supervisor. Team supervision often results in team solidarity and provides a place where greater openness and clearer feedback becomes possible (Lammers, 1999 has a very good article on team supervision).

Besides forms of supervision, there are also issues of context that affect supervision. Managerial supervision involves elements of power and authority and responsibility not usually present in developmental or reflective supervision. At times, supervisees do not feel as safe in sharing vulnerable areas. Contextual issues can also include the background in which supervisors do their work. Organisational cultural differences exist between Prison Service supervision, Probation and Social Work supervision as well as supervision in the Private Sector.

Case example

How might you respond to George in the following example?

George is an experienced Tutor on the Sex Offenders' Treatment Programme within the Prison Service. A new Treatment Manager has been appointed to oversee the programme and to supervise the two Tutors (George and Amanda). She (the Treatment Manager) is about 20 years younger than George and has had nowhere near the same experience in running the actual programme as he has had. At the first supervision meeting George suggests it might be better if he did not attend future supervision meetings. He says he has little to learn from supervision, being as experienced as he is in running the programme, and wonders how the new supervisor can supervise his work when he is more experienced in running the course than she is. He is happy for the other two to meet for supervision (Amanda, he says, is new to the programme and supervision will be of help to her).

Review and discussion

1. Outline your understanding of the essential elements in supervision. What is supervision for you?

2. Can you begin to articulate the characteristics of an effective supervisee? How do you want to use supervision?

3. At this point in your development, what form of supervision would best suit you?

4. How does the context in which you work impact on your supervision?

CHAPTER 2

The Supervisory Relationship: Choosing (or not choosing) your Supervisor

A good supervisory relationship forms the basis of effective supervision. Throughout the history of supervision, the supervisory relationship comes through as the one factor that seems to make a consistent difference in the quality of supervision and in the satisfaction of both supervisor and supervisee. If you want to know more about this, it is worth starting with Ellis (2010) who presents and evaluates the research. Hence, it is vitally important that you can engage with your supervisor in a way that facilitates your learning. Research into supervision suggests that an effective supervisor demonstrates qualities such as empathy, acceptance, flexibility, openness with confrontation, a sense of humour and appropriate self-disclosure. Whether you have engaged your supervisor's services yourself or whether that person has been given the task in your workplace, remember that you are the consumer and it is essential that your learning needs be met adequately in supervision. Having said this, we are aware that some supervisors and organisations will not see supervision as a collaborative endeavour and it is easy to be labelled 'difficult' or 'demanding' when you try to negotiate a different concept of supervision.

Most supervisees look to a supervisor to balance support with challenge so that they can benefit from new learnings without feeling undermined in the process. A supervisor, who is too accepting and supportive without also being appropriately challenging, may leave you feeling uncertain about the quality of your work. On the other hand, a supervisor who is too critical and challenging may leave you feeling unsupported, humiliated and inadequate. It is important to find in a supervisor the right balance between support and challenge, and between positive feedback and constructive critical feedback, so you are helped to move forward in your work. You may you will want to raise this topic at different times in your relationship with your supervisor.

Supervision is a unique relationship in that you and your supervisor will be discussing the wellbeing of a third person(s) who is not present. It is vital that you feel safe enough to be frank about your difficulties in order to derive the maximum benefit from the supervisory process in the interests of all concerned. Clear direct communication in supervision will enable you more easily to feed your learning back into your daily work. A supervisor with a good sense of humour can help to make the learning process a pleasure rather than a chore; humour that has a quality of sharing rather than shaming can often help us to recognise our foibles and our shortcomings without getting them out of proportion.

A short article entitled *'The Frog Prince'* (Moloney, 2005) discusses two ways to choose a coach and these methods seem equally applicable to choosing a supervisor—the *formal competitive tender* and the *'scratch and sniff'* method. The author suggests a combination of these and sees the stages for choosing your supervisor as comprising:

1. Trawling for names, getting recommendations, reviewing databases or, in many instances in organisations, the supervisors will be chosen by HR or a senior executive either individually or through the appointment of a supervision organisation.

2. Phoning potential supervisors and asking the right questions: the kinds of questions asked at this initial stage will differ depending on needs. They may include questions about qualifications, experience, background, ethical codes, etc.

3. 'Kissing the frog' (meeting the individuals). If several individual supervisors are short listed and meetings take place, then the supervisee will be looking for appropriate style, connection with the supervisor, their ability to work together.

4. Deciding—the final decision is made and a working agreement (or contract) is drawn up (see Chapter 3).

Campbell (2000) has collected a list of qualities, characteristics, features and behaviours of effective supervisors from literature, research and workshop experiences. She presents these in terms of supervisor behaviours and personal qualities—you might want to rate your supervisor on these characteristics. As you do so, remember your supervisor is human: sometimes lists like the following can be a bit unrealistic in expecting all supervisors to have all these features all the time.

Effective supervisor behaviours

1. Clarifies expectations and style of supervision.
2. Maintains consistent and appropriate boundaries.
3. Has knowledge of theory and current research.
4. Teaches practical skills.
5. Teaches case conceptualisation.
6. Provides regular and scheduled supervision.

7. Is accessible and available.
8. Encourages the exploration of new ideas and techniques.
9. Fosters autonomy.
10. Models appropriate ethical behaviour.
11. Is willing to act as a model.
12. Is personally and professionally mature.
13. Perceives growth as an ongoing model.
14. Is willing to assess the learning needs of supervisees.
15. Provides constructive criticism and feedback.
16. Is invested in the development of the supervisee.
17. Creates a relaxed learning environment.
18. Cares about the well-being of others.
19. Has the ability to be present and immediate.
20. Has an awareness of personal power.
21. Has the courage to expose vulnerabilities, make mistakes, and take risks.
22. Is non-authoritarian and non-threatening.
23. Accepts and celebrates diversity.
24. Has the ability to communicate effectively.
25. Is willing to engage in a number of learning formats (imagination, etc.).
26. Is aware of and accepts own limitations and strengths.
27. Is willing to negotiate.
28. Works collaboratively.

Personal qualities and characteristics:

1. Sense of humour.
2. Integrity.
3. People-oriented.
4. Trustworthy.
5. Honest.
6. Tenacious.
7. Open and flexible.
8. Competent.
9. Credible.
10. Considerate.

11. Respectful.
12. Understanding.
13. Sensitive.
14. Objective.
15. Congruent.
16. Tactful.
17. Genuine.
18. Curious.
19. Intelligent.
20. Warm.
21. Supportive.
22. Tolerant.
23. Encouraging.
24. Available.

Interviewing a prospective supervisor

When you are meeting up with a prospective supervisor, it is a good idea to have some questions ready. We make some suggestions here:

1. What are your qualifications and experience in supervision?
2. To which professional bodies are you affiliated?
3. What is the principal orientation in your work?
4. What is the central tenet of your supervision philosophy?
5. Do you have experience of organisational supervision? This question will pertain to supervision within an organisational context and not to all supervisors.
6. How will you expect me to prepare for supervision with you? What information will you need in advance? And what information do you want me to bring to each session?
7. Will we be able to vary our activities in supervision?
8. What are your current interests in the field?
9. Can I see an example of your supervision contract?
10. Will we have regular reviews of my progress and of our work together?
11. How do you give constructive feedback?

Questions for yourself after meeting a prospective supervisor

1. Did I feel relaxed and at ease with this person?
2. Did I have a sense that I could learn from this person?
3. Does this person possess a body of knowledge that is of interest and potential use to me?
4. Did I leave with a respect for this person's experience in the field?
5. Was I able to be honest and open with this person?
6. Did I feel satisfied with the answers to my questions?
7. Did this person have a sense of humour that I responded to positively?
8. Did I get a sense that I would receive honest feedback, both about my strengths and my areas of growth in an atmosphere of acceptance?
9. Did the person answer my questions in an open, non-defensive manner?

When you are not in a position to choose your own supervisor, you may still ask yourself the same questions and perhaps make these a basis for negotiation where possible. For example, you could request straight and honest feedback about both your strengths and weaknesses in the course of supervision. You can ask also for a reciprocal contract that allows you to give feedback about what has been useful to you and what is less useful in supervision. In this way you can set the scene for the building of a good working alliance and capitalise on what this particular professional can offer you. It is also good to ask about the person's areas of particular interest so that you can benefit from these.

You may not have an immediate answer to some of these questions—it may be an idea to see if you can negotiate to have a trial period of say, six sessions in which you can get to know one another and assess if the supervisory alliance is working well. Remember that research into supervision (as that into therapy) regularly suggests that it is the quality of the supervisory alliance that most contributes to the effectiveness of supervision. You need a space where you feel safe to bring your real concerns and where you will receive honest feedback and help. When asked by their supervisor about what they most valued in supervision, a small group of supervisees said: '*We know that you will be honest with us about our mistakes, so for that reason we really value your positive feedback too. You are not just trying to make us feel good! When we get negative feedback, it is delivered in such a way that we can hear it and we do not feel shamed or put down. If we are unsure about something it is safe to ask you to explain. It is as though it is OK to make mistakes because that is how everyone learns*'. This response reflects a balance between appropriate support and caring confrontation on the part of the supervisor and points to a good working alliance.

As mentioned above, there are times when supervisees have no say in the choice of their supervisor. Supervisors are appointed because of placements, training arrangements and practicalities in both individual and small group supervision. While this may not be a problem and may not affect the quality of the supervisory relationship or the supervision itself, it is worth taking time to look at possible implications. Sue Kaberry (1995) researched the area of abuse in supervision and interviewed fourteen supervisees who claimed their supervision was abusive in one form or another. Interestingly, nine out of the fourteen interviewees had their supervisor appointed.

We recommend when you have been allocated to a supervisor you have not chosen for yourself that you:

1. Talk about the fact that you have not chosen one another and review what it means for each of you. Supervisors too, at times, have strong feelings about this method of setting up supervisory arrangements and may need to talk about their reactions to it.

2. Look at the possible implications of this arrangement for your work together. Where supervisors have to engage in supervision as part of their overall job, they may approach the task with resentment or lack of enthusiasm or energy. Supervisees, on the other hand, can see their lack of choice as giving permission not to participate in supervision (one of us had such a supervisee who considered it was his right to be there, as required, but expected the supervisor to guide and give direction and the answers).

3. Schedule in review times to ensure there are no adverse practices entering the supervisory arena as a result of being appointed as a supervision duo or group.

4. Be specific about the expectations of each other in supervision and from organisations (if this is part of the supervisory arrangement).

This type of arrangement in supervision is akin to an arranged marriage, where couples give their consent, but may have little say in the choice of their partner. There is no reason why it may not work if both parties are prepared to talk openly about their feelings and work towards an agreed supervisory arrangement.

Codes of ethics and professional bodies

We would expect all supervisors to belong to an appropriate professional body (such as British Psychological Society, Health Care Professions Council, Association for Professional Executive Coaching and Supervision, British Association for Counselling and Psychotherapy, United Kingdom Council for Psychotherapy, CIPD, Society for Coaching Psychology) and in turn subscribe to an Ethical Framework or a Code of Ethics and Practice for Supervisors. Supervisors will not be hurt or insulted if you ask them to let you know about both of these—their Professional Body and their Code of Ethics. Many supervisors make their Code of Ethics available to supervisees. If you wanted to look at sample Codes of Ethics then you can view them at the websites of the Professional Bodies, e.g., www.bacp.com; www.emccouncil.org. and www.apecs.org. In Appendix 21 we have included a recent joint statement from four of the main professional bodies concerned with the field of Coaching around best ethical practice. You might want to have a look at that appendix before moving on and consider how this applies to your context.

Conclusion

In Chapter Two, we have highlighted the importance of your particular relationship with your supervisor—this relationship will make or break supervision for you. It cannot be stressed enough how crucial it is that you find the person best suited to facilitate your learning. Time spent on that choice is time well spent.

Case example

How might you respond to Jill in the following example?

Jill is a student on a social work course who has been appointed to Gillian as her supervisor. When asked at the first meeting what she wants from supervision, Jill replies that it is a requirement of the course that she have supervision, and so she intends to take part in it. She does not see much point in being here but if the course requires it she will participate. She indicates that she hopes it will not be too demanding and wants Gillian to tell her what to do.

Review and discussion

1. What, in your view, are the characteristics of an effective supervisor and one you would like to work with?
2. Are you in a position to choose supervision and a supervisor (even if you are appointed a supervisor)?

3. How would you know if the supervisory relationship was deteriorating?
4. How might you handle the situation if you felt the supervisory relationship was deteriorating?

CHAPTER 3

Roles and Responsibilities in Supervision

One of the areas you will notice as a prominent heading in the Supervision Contract is 'Roles and Responsibilities'. Here, we will look in some detail at your roles and responsibilities as the supervisee. First of all, there are a few areas that you need to sort out before you begin supervision. These are, as it were, the 'not negotiables' of supervision. What these are and how many they are will depend (and differ) according to your profession and your professional responsibilities.

Some of these may be:

1. Belonging to a professional body: what is the appropriate professional body to which you belong (as a trainee or a full member—professional bodies have different categories of membership)?
2. Subscribing to a professional code of ethics: usually your professed adherence to a professional code of ethics comes as part and parcel of belonging to a professional body.
3. Professional Liability Insurance for your work: such insurance is seen as more and more essential to good practice and some organisations will not employ you if you do not have this.

Other supervisee responsibilities include:

1. Your learning (objectives).
2. Applying learning from supervision.
3. Keeping notes of supervision sessions.
4. Feedback to self and to supervisor.
5. Applying learning from supervision.
6. Preparing for supervision.
7. Presenting in supervision.

We will look later at a number of these under their specific headings. Here we will concentrate on learning objectives, applying learning from supervision and keeping notes of supervision sessions.

Learning objectives

We suggest you spend time thinking through learning objectives for yourself from supervision. While overall, you take responsibility for yourself as a learning adult, here you can specify what objectives you would like to concentrate on within this supervision experience or as part of this placement.

Examples of learning objectives are:

1. To learn how to challenge clients more effectively.
2. To fine-tune my ability to make better focused, clear and energetic presentations.
3. To formulate a methodology for assessing clients.
4. To reflect on my relationship 'in the room' with this client.
5. To manage more effectively how my work with this group of clients affects me personally and professionally.
6. To work more effectively with this organisation.
7. To facilitate this team in becoming more cohesive in its relationships and its objectives.
8. To assess the next steps in my professional development.

The articulation of clear learning objectives for yourself (as well as in consultation with your supervisor) allows you to have specific end-goals towards which you are working. Agreement on learning objectives with your supervisor allows your supervisor to monitor them and give ongoing feedback on how well you are doing.

Keeping notes of supervision sessions

We recommend that you keep summary notes of your supervision sessions. During the session, it is always helpful to make notes on insights, ideas, action points and any other decisions made. This will allow you to review what happened during the supervision session and give you a summary of what action points you need to apply to your work. Keeping a 'Learning Journal' is a good idea. You can summarise your overall learning and see your supervision notes as part of such a journal.

Appendix 5 has a Supervision Recording Sheet that you might find helpful while preparing for supervision and writing up key action points and then, when preparing for your next supervision session, indicate how you have applied key concepts.

Applying learning from supervision

As a supervisee, it is your responsibility to incorporate the decisions made during supervision into your work. Having action points is often only the beginning of the process of learning. The final point of the learning curve is when you are able to implement those action points into your work. Outlining plans and ideas of how best to apply your learning to your work is a second stage.

Case example

What might you say to Jack in the following example?

Jack comes to supervision, but is very passive and quiet. In the supervision group, he only responds when contacted and does not have an agenda. He does not prepare for supervision and when asked if he has any issues he would like to bring says he does not. He takes every opportunity to absent himself from supervision. Word comes back to the supervisor that he has been heard to say that supervision is useless and he gets nothing from it.

Review and discussion

1. What learning objectives do you bring to supervision?
2. Have you a format for keeping notes of supervision sessions?
3. Can you outline your roles and responsibilities as a supervisee?
4. Are you clear about the roles and responsibilities of your supervisor?
   A. to you?
   B. to your organisation?
   C. to your placement?
   D. to your training programme?
   E. to your clients or client group?

CHAPTER 4

The Supervisory Contract

Supervision involves a number of stakeholders. For it to be effective, all stakeholders need to agree to be clear about, and subscribe to, the same objectives. Part of that planning is contracting together.

Contracts (overt and covert) underpin all relationships whether these are one-to-one, team or organisational. They contain the agreements—conscious and unconscious—of all parties in the relationship and the rules and procedures that guide these relationships. Overall, contracts revolve around:

1. *Exchange*—what we will do for each other.
2. A sense of *reciprocity*—two/multi way arrangements.
3. *Choice*—I or we freely enter this arrangement.
4. Some sense of *predictability*—we can have some guarantees that this will happen.
5. The future—we *will* do.
6. The responsibilities of parties concerned—I will take accountability for doing *x* if you take accountability for doing *y*.
7. Regular reviews.

While overt contracts attempt to articulate these elements, either verbally or in written form, words and gestures are always open to interpretation. It is because they are open to interpretation that a 'psychological contract' is part of all contracts. Individuals bring to their contracts and agreements their own assumptions, beliefs and expectations most of which will be unspoken and not negotiated. The psychological contract is the subjective side that contains our hidden agendas. This chapter will look at the importance of both types of contracts, the overt and the covert, in supervision.

Our suggestion is that you have clear and focused contracts that articulate the roles and responsibilities of all the parties involved in the supervision arrangement. We use the plural 'contracts' here because in most supervisory arrangements there will be a number of contracts and, as the central figure of supervision, you the supervisee will be involved in more than one of them.

We define the supervision contract as an agreement between supervisor and supervisee(s) about the goals of supervision. Contracting involves a two-way agreement about the focus of the supervision session to ensure that you get your needs met. Some people find the term 'contract' too formal and prefer terms like 'goal' or 'focus'. Contracts can be made to establish a focus for an individual session or for longer term, for example, to outline the overall goals for the year. We see a benefit to both types of contracting. The longer-term contract provides an overall focus to the work, and the sessional contract provides an agreed focus for an individual session.

Contracts work best if they are specific and have well-defined outcomes.

Examples are:

"What I want to do in this session is discuss the presentation that I am planning to do to verify that the ideas flow logically together and see if the sequencing and logical connection between ideas is fine. I also want to check that I am not striving to cover too much."

OR

"I want to focus on my work with a client with whom I feel a bit stuck and I'd like to decide on a way forward with the work."

You and the supervisor will negotiate the contract to ensure it is not too ambitious for the time available.

Contracts differ and there are a number of different facets to contracting in supervision. Next, briefly, we describe the different types of contracts that may be involved in the contracting process.

1. **Two-way contracts** (see Appendix 1 for an example). A two-way contract is made between the supervisee and the supervisor and is a private arrangement between them. The essence of this agreement is that the supervisee will bring his/her work to the supervisor who will provide a space for reflection and learning.

2. **Three-way contracts** (involving organisations). These contracts are three-cornered in that the agreement has three components—the supervisee, the supervisor and the organisation. These contracts may differ in degree of contact: sometimes the only contact the supervisor has with the organisation is an invoice for payment. Sometimes, however, the supervisor makes some form of report to the organisation, the

confidentiality boundaries of which needs to be stipulated clearly and understood by all three parties before the contracted work begins.

3. **The business contract** refers to the practicalities of the agreement, e.g., times, venue and length of meetings, how payments will take place and with what frequency (after each session or monthly for example), cancellation agreements, limits of confidentiality, information details required by the supervisor, copies of forms to be filled out, etc. This is the administrative aspect of the agreement.

4. **The psychological contract** refers to the agreement (on a more implicit level) that the supervisor is committed to co-creating with the supervisee a safe and facilitative environment in which work can be discussed and evaluated. It is at this level that problems often arise since the supervisor and the supervisee may have very different expectations of the process of supervision, and if these are not spelt out clearly and worked through, misunderstandings and disappointments may arise. This can, in turn, lead to 'games' and 'ruptures' in the supervisory alliance. Therefore, we encourage you at the outset to discuss carefully your expectations of supervision. We trust this manual will help you in that process. (For further reading on the psychological contract, see Carroll, 2005, *The Psychological Contract in Organisations*, where there are some exercises on how to get in touch with this elusive side of the contract). We have a section in Chapter 15 around 'critical moments' in supervision which inevitably bring up issues around trust in the supervisory relationship. You might like to have a look at that section now as a way to anticipate possible conflicts within supervision.

Managing the psychological contract

It is often the difficulties within the psychological contract that result in formal and informal complaints, legal stances and breakdowns in professional (and personal) relationships. It is imperative to look at how supervisors and supervisees can anticipate and work with this side of the contract to avoid such happenings.

Hewson (1999) has suggested ideas on managing the psychological contract in a healthy manner:

1. All parties have an active involvement in the development of the contract.

2.   The contract provides a mental set or overall perception of what end goal is in mind for everyone.

3.   Contracting creates a guard against the abuse of power and all participants are aware of and patrol the boundaries of power.

4.   Overt contracts are designed to minimise covert agendas.

5.   Transparency, honesty, openness and dialogue are built into contracting.

6.   Contracts are often developmental (they change and need to change over time, e.g., as in marriage) and need to be re-negotiated. The psychological contract is part of that development.

7.   Contracts are emotional arenas as well as rational agreements.

8.   Pay heed to the social, political, organisational and professional contexts in which contracts are lived and played out.

9.   Pick up subtle shifts in expectations from those who are part of the contract—articulate these expectations.

10. Track the relationships to see if any new needs emerge (e.g., that the supervisee might need more support or counselling).

Contracts have been compared by Proctor (2008) to Russian Dolls. There are contracts within contracts and these can take place between different parties within the overall supervisory/training system:

1.   there is the overall contract between the two participants and the organisation (e.g., training establishment);

2.   within that is the contract between the individual supervisee and the organisation;

3.   within 2 there is the supervisory contract between the supervisor and supervisee;

4.   these, and the other contracts, need to be aligned so that all are agreed on what will happen.

There is also an ongoing process of contracting that supports the supervision process. This involves the overall learning contract you make with your supervisor that stipulates your learning goals for supervision over the time of your contact with the supervisor. This contract covers your 'growing edges' or areas for development so that both you and the supervisor are clear about what your work together will entail.

Within this larger contract, you will then also contract session-by-session regarding your needs and goals for that particular session. These sessional contracts will help you to keep focused on your learning needs. Contracting can also be used as a relational tool within the session so that you can make mini-contracts when you want more or less of something, or when a need or area of interest arises in the course of a session and you want to change direction. The use of contracting in this way means that you and your supervisor can keep track of your goals in an ongoing way and not get sidetracked into something that is not useful to you.

Connor and Pokora (2007) list a number of items that they suggest considering as part of a working agreement.

Practical

1. Having a pre-supervisory introductory session.
2. Agreement on a location—where will you meet?
3. Frequency—how often will you be meeting? Minimum/maximum number of sessions.
4. Length of session—what would you prefer? Agree to?
5. Payment—how much? Payment procedure?
6. Cancellation—policy for missed session? What if the supervisee is late?

Working relationship

1. Preferred ways of working together.
2. Tools and techniques you might use.
3. Your values and the learning relationship.
4. Balance of support and challenge you might offer.
5. Feedback—discuss the nature of feedback.
6. How the supervisee learns best?
7. Framework or model you use
8. Your expectations—work outside of sessions.

Professional

1. Your qualifications.
2. Your experience/references.
3. Your responsibilities: legal, to the supervisee, to your profession, to the organisation.
4. Any possible conflicts of interest?
5. Note-taking: who takes? Who keeps? For how long?
6. Supervision—your arrangements.

Ethical

1. An explicit working agreement.
2. Built-in ongoing review.
3. Confidentiality: extent and limits.
4. Clear role boundaries.
5. Ending session.

Managing confidentiality

A crucial part of the supervision partnership, and an essential ingredient in all the above contracts, is an agreed understanding of what 'confidentiality' means to all parties concerned. When it is not clear (and unfortunately at times even when it has been agreed) leakage of information can take place when so many players are concerned—the organisation, the managers, HR, the helping company, the individual's supervisor, the training organisation, the supervisee himself or herself, and other stakeholders or participants. Steps need to be taken, before supervision begins, to set up a confidentiality structure so that all stakeholders are clear about what is agreed.

There are four types of confidentiality and it is important to know which type is being considered in supervision and not assume there is automatic agreement on what confidentiality means. The four types are:

1. *Absolute confidentiality* is an agreement where under no circumstances would confidentiality be broken, no matter what information was discussed or revealed. The most obvious example of absolute confidentiality is the Roman Catholic confessional. It would also seem to pertain for solicitors and barristers who have 'privileged information'. Often supervisees think that absolute confidentiality is being offered when it is not, but because of lack of clarity they can get upset and angry if disclosure needs to take place with or without their permission.

2. *Limited confidentiality* agrees that what is discussed and shared between parties will be confidential with agreed exceptions to that rule, e.g., one of us worked with an oil company where knowledge of alcohol or drug abuse on the oil rigs had to be fed back to the Company. It was written into the agreement and all parties were aware of this. Other common instances of limited confidentiality are: where there is serious danger to self or others, or child abuse and other harmful activities. However, please note that all

citizens in the United Kingdom are legally bound to disclose confidential information if it involves terrorism or drug money laundering. What is excluded from being confidential varies in relation to context, but what is important is that all parties are aware of these conditions and agree to them before supervision commences.

3. *Discretionary confidentiality* is where supervisees or clients leave it to the discretion of the supervisor where and when to use the information that emerges from their supervisory sessions. This is a very trusting attitude; this model worked well in a situation where one of us ran a youth counselling service in London. Many young people (not all indeed) would give the counsellor permission to use whatever they needed in the welfare and help of the young person himself or herself.

4. *Negotiated confidentiality* is a form of confidentially that can cover any or all of the above (and will pertain in all situations) but where the participants start with a blank sheet of paper and work out the type of confidentially that best suits them. This will involve discussions with and about how to involve/or not, other stakeholders in the supervisory arrangement. However, the negotiation will also reflect individual needs and circumstances.

Our suggestion is that the norm in supervision will be 'limited confidentiality' where it is clear about where, when and to whom disclosures are made.

Case example

How might you discuss the following with the supervisees?

With the new Tutors on the Training Programme, you discuss the possibility of a supervision contract. This is the first time you have supervised them, even though both are experienced supervisees. They look surprised when you mention the word 'contract' and after a few moments silence, they react quite negatively. They have not had supervision contracts before, they tell you, and they don't see much point in having one. Don't you trust them, they want to know. They tell you they are fearful that if they sign a contract it may be held against them at some later date.

Review and discussion

1. What are the features of an effective contract?
2. Do you think you are now able to negotiate a supervisory contract with your supervisor?

3. What might you do if your supervisor is not interested in negotiating or even having a contract?

4. What part will the psychological contract play in your overall contract with your supervisor? With the organisation? With the training establishment?

CHAPTER 5

Preparing for Supervision

Careful preparation for supervision is one of the best 'insurance policies' for it to work well. Effective preparation entails having a clear method of preparation and a way to ensure you bring to supervision what you most need to learn. Some areas worthy of review are:

1. Am I inclined to bring only my problems to supervision?
2. Do I bring only my good work to supervision?
3. Do I balance what I bring to supervision between what I consider my good work and my poor work?
4. Am I aware there are aspects of my work that I would prefer not to bring to supervision?
5. Am I hiding some parts of my work from my supervisor? Have I in the past? Why?
6. Do I carefully edit what I bring to supervision in order to avoid potential or feared shame and embarrassment?

Answers to these questions will help you think through, openly and honestly, how you prepare for supervision.

Preparation is the 'before' of supervision, the time spent when I think through, reflect on, sift and decide on my agenda for supervision. Some requirements for being able to do this are:

1. Time set aside for preparation.
2. Creating an environment of reflection, honesty and openness with oneself.
3. Recall of work (using your notes or recordings from your work).
4. Creating an agenda (prioritising).

Here are some methods you could use to help your preparation:

1. Listening to recordings/viewing videos of your work.
2. Process recordings.
3. Team preparation/small group preparation.
4. Keeping a learning journal.

Getting ready for supervision

As you prepare for your supervision session and organise your agenda it is worth focusing on what you want from the session. One way is to see if you can distinguish between the following:

1. **A puzzle:** something I can resolve that is confusing to me just now and for which there is an answer that would apply to most situations and people, e.g., how to answer the phone in a more facilitative manner. A puzzle has one right answer.

2. **A problem:** again what is solvable, but the solution will change from person to person and from situation to situation, e.g., my relationship with my boss; my relationship with a particular client. There is an answer to a problem, but each person has to find his or her own particular answer.

3. **A paradox:** something that cannot be solved but with which I have to learn to live, e.g. that I am going to be made redundant and would prefer not to be, that my father has died and I am not sure how I can live without him and still practice as a therapist.

4. **A psychological problem:** a problem that keeps recurring, e.g., all my relationships with my male bosses end up in fights; I have problems with all my female tutors on the course. This is a recurring and repetitive pattern.

5. **A mystery:** events that happen in life that are difficult or impossible for me to make sense of, e.g., Why do I have cancer when I have done nothing wrong to deserve it? At what stage do I accept that I can no longer do this job? If there is a God why does he allow suffering? Why must we die?, etc.

Each of the above needs a different intervention for resolution: hence the importance of knowing what you are dealing with.

The menu for supervision

A question beginning supervisees often have is about the areas covered by supervision. What is the subject matter of supervision? What is supervision about in terms of content areas? In short, what is on the supervision menu? One way to think about the supervision menu is in terms of the five *'Bands of Supervision'* offered by Clarkson and Gilbert (1991) that can be the focus in any supervision session. Most sessions concentrate on one (or two) bands at most in terms of the supervisee's priorities.

The bands of supervision

1. Assessment and treatment planning.
2. Strategies and intervention techniques.
3. Parallel process.
4. Theory (teaching and integration).
5. Ethics and professional practice.

We will briefly describe each of these bands.

Assessment and treatment planning

This band focuses on the question: How to think about the situation?

Understanding the parameters of the client or group's problem before moving on may be necessary as a first step. This band involves questions of client assessment, clear definitions of problems and thinking of an overall plan for working with a particular problem over time. How do you foresee that this process may unfold and what are the potential problem areas to anticipate at each stage? There is plenty of interesting material in the literature on stages of treatment planning in therapy or on stages of group development that can assist you in planning and avoiding some potential problems. In this way, you can benefit from the wisdom of others already in the field before you and use their experience as a guide.

Strategies and intervention techniques

This band focuses on the question: What to do about the situation?

Here the discussion focuses on possible techniques and strategies that will achieve a particular goal/s. Sometimes as a supervisee you may be 'stuck' with a particular client, team or client group and feel you have reached an impasse. Working out practical strategies to take you forward may be most helpful to you at this stage. If you can bring an audio recording that illustrates the actual 'stuck point', your supervisor will be able to help you more effectively. Supervisees may also come to supervision with a desire to broaden their range of interventions and techniques so they can add something new to their repertoire. This may involve learning a 'two-chair' technique, refining skills in empathic transactions, practicing phenomenological enquiry, or acquiring some group intervention skills, etc.

Parallel process (reflection of the transference/counter transference dynamic)

This band focuses on the question: What is going on in the supervision situation?

Sometimes the very problem the client has brought to the counsellor is played out in supervision. For example, a client may 'overwhelm' a counsellor with a wealth of information so that it is impossible to take it in rapidly, and the counsellor may then 'pour out' to the supervisor all this information and repeat the very process that she is struggling with in the client sessions. This is called 'parallel process' and enables the supervisor to work with this process with the supervisee in a live 'here-and-now' way in the supervisory session. Or the client may complain of feeling helpless, and the supervisee will bring her own feelings of helplessness and inadequacy to the supervisor. Such parallel process dynamics can be focused on effectively in supervision with a view to finding a way forward in the client work. In a similar manner, the transference issues brought by the client (for example, mistrust of the therapist based on earlier mistrust of a parent figure) can form an important part of a supervision session. The therapist's own response to the client (counter transference) can provide a fertile ground for discussion related to areas where the supervisee 'gets hooked' by clients and/or in providing valuable information about how this client impacts other people.

Often when supervisees 'get stuck' with a client it is the counter transference response that is blocking them rather than a lack of technique!

Theory (teaching and integration)

This band focuses on the question: What information is lacking in the situation?

Supervisees may desire information about a particular area of work or a problem area with which they are unfamiliar. A supervisee might be working with a group of clients about whom he/she will have little prior knowledge (for example, clients with eating disorders or drug problems). The supervisee may then turn to the supervisor for theoretical and clinical information and want to be pointed to sources of reading and support. There may also be a request to integrate new information into the supervisee's ongoing practice and to get help relating new aspects of theory to practice and integrating these into the supervisee's style of working. We see the task of 'teaching' very much as part of the supervision process (see also Carroll, 1996 on the seven tasks of supervision).

Ethics and professional practice

This band focuses on the question: What should happen in the situation?

Sometimes the supervisee is faced with an ethical dilemma or an issue related to professional practice, all of which is most fruitfully talked over in supervision so that a way forward can be decided. This may involve an ethical issue related to confidentiality, to dual relationships or to requests for information from solicitors—the supervisee may need guidance about how to proceed. Ethics involves principles rather than rules so it is part of professional development to grow into ethical thinking about situations you may face. There is not usually an easy answer! Professional issues involve our relationships with our professional peers and often involve disagreements and conflicts about differing views of practice and conduct towards other professionals. In our experience, such problems are brought more and more frequently to supervision as the profession develops and expands. (See Appendix 4 for a model of ethical decision making for supervisees).

Confidentiality will be a part of any supervisory contract just as it is when we see clients. It is essential that confidentiality be maintained with regard to the material discussed, ensuring a safe holding environment for all concerned. However, confidentiality is seldom absolute and this needs to be clear to all concerned.

1. Most ethics codes stipulate that confidentiality may be broken if the client or others in his/her environment are at risk. In such a case, the supervisor's support will be essential.

2. If you work in an organisational context, then that organisation may have its own parameters about confidentiality and it is important that you know these. For example, if you are counselling in a bank, then you may be obliged to report cases of fraud if these are disclosed to you. It is your duty to acquaint yourself with the codes of practice of the particular organisation in which you work and make sure that clients also understand these.

3. Anyone in this country (and most other countries for that matter) is under an obligation to assist the police in cases of 'treason' or 'terrorism' so confidentiality agreements cannot legally cover these areas. Check your code of ethics or organisational policies and procedures to ensure you know and have a clear understanding of what comes under, and what does not, the areas of confidentiality, e.g., issues of child protection.

4. You need to make it clear to clients that you receive supervision and that you will be taking confidential material to your supervisor who is bound by a code to keep this confidential. Where realistic, it is good to add that you will not reveal any names and distinguishing details (as far as possible).

As we mentioned above, a particular supervision session may involve one (or at the most two) of these bands of supervision. A knowledge of the bands, however, will give you some idea of common areas brought to supervision and therefore enable you to prepare your questions more effectively in advance of the session.

What is permissible to bring to supervision?

Supervision covers areas related to your practice as a professional. These may range from a challenge you are facing with a client to getting help with becoming self-employed, or from resolving how much to charge for your services to liaising and networking with other professionals. It might revolve around seeking help with where and how to advertise your services. Supervision is to assist you in becoming a more effective professional in all ways!

When we speak to new supervisees about what to bring to supervision we say that supervision is about any issue that impinges on your professional life and may cause you difficulties at present in your work. What that is will be influenced greatly by the contexts in which supervisees work. However, the areas covered could include personal life changes or interpersonal difficulties that affect your quality of work. The above question relates to any of the areas covered by the bands of supervision, but here we particularly wish to raise the issue of personal problems/issues that may influence your work with a client/s. This raises the question of the interface between therapy/counselling and supervision. If an issue affects you in the workplace, then it may be important to mention it in supervision. Examples may include concerns about your health, problems in your partnership that affect your confidence, a family bereavement that has deeply affected you, a query about a change of career, etc. These may also include relationship conflicts with peers or bosses.

The supervisor's role is to make sense with you of the implications of the issue for your work with clients and to help you to think about effective support for yourself. The more deep-seated personal aspects of the problem would fall into the realm of therapy/counselling, but the impact of the issue on your working life can be a supervision issue. Your supervisor is part of your professional support network and can also help you to review what other supports may be important to set in place for yourself.

Hawkins and Shohet (2000) outline a process model of supervision that has seven focus areas of what supervisees can bring to supervision. Inskipp and Proctor (2001) renamed this model *'The Seven-Eyed Supervisor'*. The seven focus points are:

1. Clients (individuals, groups, organisations) that are the focus of our work.
2. Interventions—what are we doing to bring about a difference?
3. Relationships—what kind of relationship is involved and is it working?
4. Reactions—what is happening to the supervisee as he/she is doing the work?
5. What is happening between supervisor and supervisee? Does this reflect in any way what is happening between supervisee and their work?
6. What is happening to the supervisor as he or she listens and works with what is brought to supervision?
7. What organisational issues are having an impact on the work?

In our view, all these focal points are valid and permissible areas for supervision and all will impact on the actual work of the supervisee for the benefit of the client which, of course, is the main and central discussion point of supervision.

Exercise

Have your notebook beside you. Relax, take some deep breaths and allow yourself to concentrate on your breathing for a minute or two. Then let your mind drift back over your recent work (programmes delivered, individual work, etc.).

What immediately surfaces for you? Notice it and let it go (you might want to make a note of it in your supervision notebook). Let your mind wander over the following questions:

1. What interactions/sessions/clients/interventions were you pleased with?
2. What was difficult for you?
3. What were you/are you uncertain about?
4. What are you looking forward to in your next working session?
5. Are there any anxieties about the way you are working with a particular client/group/programme?
6. Are there any anxieties about your relationship with clients/other tutors/ managers, etc?
7. Are there some doubts/anxieties/feelings just 'out of view' that you would rather keep out of view? Identify the feelings as well as the items.
8. What interactions have you enjoyed most? What were the feelings?

Jot down a list of what has surfaced for you as a result of this reverie.

Scan through your records/notes. Do any further points stand out that you would like/need to talk about? Add to your list.

Imagine you are replaying a video of one session (or part of one). Are there any ideas or feelings that come up for you which you, might, or might not, like to bring to your supervisor? Note them.

Read through your list. Mark with an 'N' any items that do not seem significant enough to bring to supervision just now, mark with a 'P' any items you feel reluctant to talk about, would rather postpone (there may not be any). Tentatively prioritise the remaining items by numbering Item, 1, 2, 3, etc.

If you have marked some 'P' items, gently explore with yourself what the risks would be to you, or to your relationship with your supervisor, if you to bring these up? What might you gain/learn if you did?

Think about what you want to learn from this session of supervision and how you might present your material.

Immediate preparation for the supervisory session:

1.   Are there any crisis/emergency issues you need to talk about?
2.   Are there any themes emerging for you in your overall work you would like to review in supervision?
3.   Are there any organisational/training areas you want to talk about in supervision?
4.   What do you want from this session of supervision? For yourself, your clients, your learning?
5.   Are there any areas of the supervisory contract you want to review/re-negotiate?

(Adapted from Inskipp & Proctor, 2001).

Another way to prepare for supervision is to use the *Seven Eyes of Supervision* (mentioned above) and presented in Appendix 7.

Case example

How might you respond to the supervisee in the following example?

Peter says in his supervision group that he wants to discuss his working relationship with a colleague who is in difficulties. When the supervisor asks how he would describe the difficulty, Peter replies in general terms and with some irritation in his voice: he says he wants to 'get on with it' and 'this is not helpful'. He tells his story and the supervisor and group members get involved in a long and detailed discussion with Peter of the events of the past few weeks that have generated the 'difficulty'. After half an hour, the supervisor draws the discussion to a close since others want time to present. At this point Peter says: "I feel even more confused now than I did when I arrived. I still do not know how to approach my colleague when I see her again". Everyone in the group feels disappointed.

Review and discussion

1. Do you a have a clear method for preparing for supervision?
2. What are the factors in your life that interfere, just now, with your preparation time?

CHAPTER 6

Presenting in Supervision

Supervisees create the supervision agenda. They bring their concerns, joys, worries, problems and celebrations to supervision sessions. In preparation, they organise and prioritise what they want from supervision. In presenting their material in supervision, they want to use the time economically and beneficially.

A good place to start thinking about the presentation of material in supervision is by answering some of these questions:

1. Why am I bringing this to supervision?
2. What am I hoping for from supervision/supervisor/other supervisees in respect to this area?

There are a number of ways of presenting your work in supervision:

Verbally

I present my work orally to the supervisor.

I can 'tell the story' of a particular client or client session or describe an event that I wish to review with my supervisor. In this case I may rely on some notes or on my memory. This can be useful when an overview of a situation or a client's life story is necessary to put a problem or my question in context.

Notes

I give my notes in advance to my supervisor.

I can prepare notes of a session or a problem or an area for discussion and let my supervisor have these in advance so that he/she can read them before the session. This may be useful when I am preparing a presentation or a written case study or writing a letter to another professional that I wish to review first.

Audio and video

Playing audio or video sections of a session with a client or a presentation or a team meeting will give my supervisor a very alive 'here-and-now' sense of the process I wish to discuss. The advantage of this method is that I do not rely entirely on my memory or my notes but have the actual words and interventions available for review. This is especially useful if I feel 'stuck' and want to look at alternative interventions or explore my own responses to the client/situation. Recordings allow for a detailed intervention-by-intervention analysis of my work. Since they can be rewound and played many times over, they allow the supervisee to listen anew to his/her interventions and try out new responses. Campbell (2000) has a section in her book (Appendix C, p. 261) where she outlines some instructions for audio and video recordings. These include:

1. Use quality equipment.
2. Buy good quality tapes or a reliable recording device.
3. Where you place the equipment matters.
4. Check background sound and volume.
5. Know how to use the equipment before you begin.
6. Protect the confidentiality of client and supervisee.
7. Process any anxiety and concern with client (and with yourself as supervisee) before recording.
8. Explain recording, its goals and purposes to the client at least one session before proceeding.
9. Get a written Release Form from the client, i.e., written permission to record sessions declaring who will have access to the recording.
10. Before beginning the actual session, check the equipment one more time!

Process reports

You can also write up a process report after a session or a meeting and take this to supervision. The advantage is that the supervisor will get a sense of the ongoing process that you went through as well as the moment-by-moment interventions in the context of the whole session. Such a process report could be augmented with a brief audio recording of a central section of the session. Process reports are particularly useful in contexts in which recording is either not possible or not permitted.

Knapman and Morrison (1998) point out that process recording is a way of:

'Recording in detail either during the interview or immediately afterwards what was said by both parties, recording the non-verbal cues given by both parties and any analysis of what you, the supervisee, thought might be happening. Useful triggers can be sections entitled:

1. *what I said;*
2. *what he/she said;*

3. *what I felt;*
4. *what I told myself;*
5. *what I did;*
6. *what he/she/they did;*
7. *what seemed to be happening at this point.'*

See Appendix 6: Horton, I. (1993). Supervision. In R. Bayne & P. Nicolson (Eds.), *Counselling and Psychology for Health Professionals* (pp. 28–31). London: Chapman and Hall.

Keeping notes of supervision sessions

We recommend that you keep summary notes of your supervision sessions. During the session, it is always helpful to make notes on insights, ideas, action points and any other decisions made. This will allow you to review what happened during supervision and give you a summary of what action points you need to apply to your work. Keeping a 'Learning Journal' is a good idea. In it you can summarise your overall learning and see your supervision notes as part of such a journal.

As a supervisee, it is your responsibility to incorporate the decisions made during supervision into your work. Having action points is often only the beginning of the process of learning. The final point of the learning curve is when you are able to implement those action points into your work. Outlining plans and ideas of how best to apply your learning to your work is a second stage.

Appendix 15 on the Learning Log has a format to help you capture learnings from your supervisory session. Have a look at it now and consider if it might help if you fill it in after your sessions.

Case example

How might you manage John's reaction in the following?

One of the supervisees in your small group regularly does not keep to the manual. When you have confronted him in the group he points out that the manual is only a guideline and what is needed is creative work in the 'here-and-now'. You suspect he is too lazy to really prepare. But he is a strong individual and you can see that he has an effect on other supervisees who are beginning to take a lead from him. You are wondering how you can put this on the agenda for supervision without causing too much conflict.

Review and discussion

1. What is the best way for you to present effectively in supervision?
2. What are the pros and cons of different methods of presentation in supervision?

CHAPTER 7

Understanding Developmental Stages of Learning in Supervision

Identifying your own learning style will be an advantage in terms of identifying what helps you most effectively in supervision. However, before we do this, it may be helpful to reflect on the overall process of learning over time that occurs through the effective use of good supervision. We will outline these stages briefly here.

Stage 1: Relying on your own internal critic as supervisor

In our experience as supervisors, we have noticed a tendency in supervisees when they first come to supervision to use their own internal critics as 'supervisors'. They often judge themselves and their work very harshly and in a global manner. For example, supervisees may say of themselves: *"You see I never get anything right"*, or *"There I go again, stupid as always"*, or *"I constantly make a mess of things"*, or *"I am no good at conflict resolution"*. Such global statements can be damning of you and your work and do not leave you any room for improvement. Statements like those often form part of an internal dialogue, i.e., internal critics based on our earlier experiences with significant people, or simply opinions of ourselves that have never been checked out in a supportive environment where we can receive realistic feedback.

Because we may have been shamed or humiliated for 'not knowing' when we were younger, we may quite understandably have grown reluctant to reveal our lack of knowledge or our need for help in any particular area of work. Good supervision provides an opportunity to undo this harmful reticence and provides us with a place where we can truly learn what we want to know! So it may be a good start to identify the unhelpful messages from your own 'internal critic' and challenge these for yourself and/or discuss them with your supervisor and your peers.

This first stage thus marks a move from *'unconscious incompetence to conscious incompetence'* (Robinson, 1974): you get to realise what you do not know in your particular area of work. This can, at best, result in a realistic setting of learning goals as you identify the areas you need to learn and refine. Sometimes this process of becoming aware of what you still have to learn may leave you feeling deskilled, so it is important to remind yourself that this is a natural part of learning anything new.

Stage 2: The stage of the 'internalised' supervisor

We are indebted to Casement (1985) for the concepts of the *'internalised supervisor'* and the *'internal supervisor'*. In the process of interacting with a supervisor you will gradually move from drawing on your own internal critic to drawing on the wisdom and experience of your supervisor. In this process you will introject or take into your own internal mental world your real life supervisor's attitudes and ideas. In practical terms this means using the wisdom and suggestions of your supervisor to support your work. This stage is often marked by the supervisee following the advice of a supervisor very literally, and even using his/her very words in working with people.

This may seem to some of you to represent an over-reliance on your supervisor but we see this as a natural stage of the learning process as you gradually allow the ideas of someone else to impact on you and assist you in your work. Supervisees at this stage may say to the supervisor: *"I could hear your voice in my head"* or *"I remembered your words as I sat opposite the person I discussed in supervision last time we met"*. This marks the process of *'internalising the supervisor'* and gradually replacing the critic in your head, who may have been undermining you rather than helping you to learn, with an image of your supervisor. At this stage it is also important to feel your supervisor acknowledges your experience and supports your ongoing development and evolving personal style of working.

This stage marks the movement from *'conscious incompetence to conscious competence'* (Robinson, 1974) as you gradually internalise new knowledge and new skills. These may still seem a little foreign to you as you may take these on in an undigested way from your supervisor or from other sources of learning. However, you need to take in new ideas and skills before you can fully digest these and make them your own. For each of us, imitation can be a very effective means of learning something new and difficult.

Stage 3: Developing your own 'internal supervisor'

At this stage as a supervisee, you begin to develop your own 'internal supervisor' that integrates what has been learnt from your supervisor and everything from your own reflections, experimenting, observations and reading. It is a process of developing your own criteria for good practice and being able to judge for yourself when you are being effective or ineffective in your work. At this stage a person is in the process of developing or refining his/her own personal style of working which may in some ways resemble your supervisor's style but will have your own unique personal stamp. At this stage you will digest what you have learned and you will change or retain individual elements that suit your style as a person and as a professional.

What we consider important at this stage is that as a supervisee you can own your own competence and assess the quality of your work by realistic standards. One of the important processes in developing effective work habits is relinquishing the idea that there is only one right way of doing things and, instead, consider how we can be as effective as possible in a certain context. This stage marks the move from *'conscious competence to unconscious competence'* (Robinson, 1974) as we gradually integrate what we know and begin to practice our art and skills without constant vigilance and hesitation. The danger at this point is that you may become a bit too relaxed; so supervision remains an important part of staying in touch with yourself and your work.

Questions to assess whether I am moving from one stage to another

From Stage 1 to Stage 2

1. Am I beginning to challenge myself when I get frustrated because I feel that I am 'not doing things right' and am focusing instead on whether my actions are getting the desired result or not?
2. Is the 'noise' in my head lessening and being replaced by a more supportive voice that allows me to make mistakes?
3. Am I asking for what I really want in supervision or am I still avoiding bringing my mistakes and difficulties?
4. Do I now have a clear idea of my learning goals so that these are in line with my stage of professional development and clearly known by the supervisor and me?
5. Am I making effective contracts with my supervisor so that I am getting all of my learning needs met in supervision?

From Stage 2 to Stage 3

1. Am I beginning to feel more confident about my own decisions when working?
2. Am I setting realistic and achievable goals in my work and enjoying the satisfaction of reaching these?
3. Do I feel empowered in supervision to explore my own thinking and feelings about situations?

4.   Do I allow my supervisor to 'give' to me and share his/her wisdom, or am I not really open to this process?

5.   Am I gradually developing my own internal criteria for effectiveness so that I am no longer so dependent on the judgement of my supervisor?

Stage 3 onwards…

1.   Do I have clear criteria by which to assess my own work?

2.   Am I able to judge when I do something well? When I make a mistake, can I remedy it without plunging into shame?

3.   Do I generally trust my own judgement, thinking and capacity to make effective choices in my work setting?

4.   Do I know when I need help or support? Can I ask for this openly and honestly?

5.   Am I taking steps to maintain a lively interest in my work by exploring new facets and ideas that engage my interest?

One of the best books on this subject is *IDM Supervision: An Integrated Developmental Model of Supervision* (Stoltenberg & McNeill, 2010). It contains a Supervisee Questionnaire to help supervisees understand their level of development and draws out the various tasks faced by supervisees at the three different levels of development.

Transference and counter transference in supervision

Transference is usually understood to refer to attitudes, feelings and unresolved issues that we bring from the past into our current relationships that influence good contact in the present. Counter transference would then refer to similar attitudes and feelings on the part of the supervisor that interfere with his/her capacity to really see and meet the supervisee. If we are both carrying 'baggage' from the past into the present, especially if this is out of our awareness, then we are unlikely to have a real meeting in the present. It is as though we will be experiencing one another through the lens of the past.

Transference is a likely occurrence in supervision and can sometimes be readily identified. Often this transference is related to other authority figures from our past with whom we have had conflicts; these unresolved feelings are then projected onto the supervisor and we may have difficulty separating out what belongs to the present and what to the past. This can lead to feelings of anger or resentment that may or may not have any basis in the present but will be seen by others as an overreaction to an event. Not all anger is transference! The distinction is about whether it seems appropriate to the present event or not! However, it may also happen that the supervisor reminds us of someone we revered in the past, and then this idealisation is projected on to the present supervisor. This may place a heavy burden on the supervisor to be like someone he/she has never met rather than being himself/herself in the relationship! Such feelings of idealisation can help the working alliance to develop but a more realistic picture of the actual person will gradually need to emerge for you if the relationship is to survive and not end in disappointment. For the supervisor too, counter transference may be a help or a hindrance in developing a good working alliance. If you have a sense that the supervisor is not really 'seeing you' then it would be a good idea to raise that matter and discuss your relationship openly so that it is based more realistically in the present.

Questions to ask yourself about transference. In the presence of my supervisor:

1. Do I feel 'small' and 'vulnerable'?
2. Do I experience similar feelings to what I have experienced with other authority figures in my life such as parents or teachers?
3. Do I feel very much in awe of my supervisor?
4. Am I prone to feelings of shame in the supervision session?
5. Am I scared to ask for what I really need?
6. Do I feel as though I have a 'crush' on him/her (the supervisor)?
7. Do I silence myself?

Identifying the transferential feelings will help you to recognise and manage them better as they arise. You may even make this recognition a part of the supervision contract with an agreement that you will not allow these feelings to disempower you and prevent you from getting your learning needs met. Clear open communication about needs and feelings is the best way through to a more effective working alliance.

Dealing with my 'drivers' in supervision

The concept of 'drivers' derives from Transactional Analysis (Kahler, 1974, 1978) and refers to ways in which we take on common 'parental' messages from our culture and then use these to push, drive and berate ourselves. Essentially a driver is our translation of a message meant to help us work more effectively but that we have turned instead into a stick with which to beat ourselves! We speak of 'driver' behaviour as having a driven quality to it because it is lacking in spontaneity and creativity. It is essentially compulsive behaviour that does not allow for reflection and imagination but drives us ever onward to do things rather than to pause to 'be' fully in the present. We will review here the common 'drivers' in our culture and as you read these you can check whether any of them hold any power for you.

The 'be perfect' driver

People with this 'driver' are constantly pushing themselves to do things 'perfectly' without any mistakes. They can often get stuck because they are trying to get a particular detail (for example, the opening sentence to a document) 'just right' and so may never get to finish a job. They may have been told *"If a thing is worth doing, it is worth doing it well"*, which is eminently good advice but has become translated into having everything 'perfect'—an impossible goal in an imperfect world! All drivers contain an element of good advice, in this case that an attention to detail is important in many jobs. However, it is the compulsive attempt to perfect everything before moving on that constitutes this 'driver' behaviour.

In this person's world there are to be no mistakes; and the idea that we may learn from our mistakes and experiments is anathema to them. They want to get it right the first time as if there is never going to be another chance to correct their mistakes. In fact, they believe you only have one chance at things and if you miss this then it is the end! They also use the words 'right' and 'wrong' frequently as though there is a perfectly 'right' way of doing everything. You can already hear what pressure this may place on a person and how little room it leaves for learning from our mistakes. This supervisee will be so focused on 'getting it right' that he/she may not get any of his/her own actual learning needs met in supervision because they are focused on 'doing supervision right'!

The 'please others' driver

This 'driver' involves the person in over-adapting to the needs and demands of others while sacrificing his/her own. This person is compulsively pleasing and struggles when anyone is displeased with him/her or any aspect of his/her behaviour. They want to be 'liked' at all costs even if this requires foregoing their own needs and demands in a situation. Of course, it is important in any work context that we can co-operate with others and consider their needs and demands in an adult and considerate manner. Teamwork is essential to good functioning at work and to be a good team member does require some accommodation to others. It is the driven nature of the 'please others' driver that leaves this person little space or time to consider his/her own needs and desires in any situation. They struggle with displeasing others and will avoid conflict at all costs even if they suffer as a result.

A person with a 'please others' driver will have over-adapted to parental figures in childhood and these patterns can be very persistent. In supervision, this supervisee will try to second-guess what the supervisor 'wants' and will work out how to please the supervisor rather than focusing on his/her own learning needs.

The 'try hard' driver

People with this driver often believe that everything in life is difficult and that they will struggle with whatever they undertake. They may have a frown on their faces regularly and talk about their struggles, seldom focusing on achievements or completed tasks. As children these people have often received the message that they will struggle but not achieve success so they are left believing there is virtue in trying hard even if they never succeed at anything. They will not allow themselves space to play and be creative and imaginative as though those processes are forbidden. They may also focus unhelpfully on mistakes and not accept them as an opportunity for learning but regard them instead as irreparable fault-lines in their characters and inevitable for a people like themselves. They will bring this struggle to supervision and find it hard to learn anything new without regarding their lack of knowledge as some basic character flaw in themselves. The biggest challenge for this person is to begin to experience learning as fun and to realise and enjoy successes.

The 'be strong' driver

This person believes in keeping a 'stiff upper lip' and not admitting to any vulnerability or need for dependence on others. The central belief is that it is important to be strong at all times in all situations; to 'cope on my own' rather than needing anything from others or in any way depending on them for assistance. Of course, some degree of independence and self-reliance is important in a work context but a compulsive persistence to be strong when you need help and could receive this readily from others is the hallmark of this 'be strong driver' behaviour. Again, it is the compulsive nature of the behaviour that interferes with effective functioning. This person will have particular difficulty in bringing any vulnerabilities, mistakes or needs to supervision believing that the supervisor will see this as a source of weakness and incompetence. Permission to get it wrong and bring mistakes to supervision is crucial to the person with the 'be strong' driver.

The 'hurry up' driver

The person with this driver behaviour is always in a hurry and will never pause or take things slowly. Time for reflection, for play and for creative thinking is often regarded as a waste of time. Of course, there are times when doing a job speedily and efficiently are really vital to the success of a task. However, the person with the 'hurry up' driver will be rushing all the time often at the cost of doing things carefully and allowing time for revision or checking for mistakes. This person was often not allowed to move at his/her own pace as a child and so learnt to rush at everything in order to avoid chastisement. This driven compulsive pattern can become really counterproductive in situations where a more measured and careful approach will get better results.

The person with this driver often comes to supervision with a list that he/she hurries through, not leaving much time for discussion, reflection or imaginative play. This makes learning a chore to be completed rather than an enjoyable and creative process. He/she will struggle if slowed down to reflect and generate different options and ideas although this is really the permission he most needs from the supervisor, for example, permission to carry some less urgent matters over to the next session!

Most of us do not just possess one driver but may manifest a combination of these in a hierarchy of importance. For example, we may please others by being perfect and try hard to be strong! You have probably realised by now that these compulsive driver behaviours are the opposite of creative, spontaneous, playful learning. They all add an element of pressure into work and supervision that interferes fundamentally with our competence, enjoyment and effectiveness.

See the Drivers Checklist in Appendix 14.

Getting it wrong

We are devoting a separate section to the idea of 'getting it wrong' because we so often meet supervisees who believe there is only one 'right' way to do something and that if they do not find it they are somehow inferior or inadequate!

We substitute the idea of effective outcomes for 'getting it right' so that people start evaluating what they do in terms of the goals they set themselves rather than feeling caught in a right/wrong dynamic. Many people who come to us for training and supervision have had the experience of an educational system in which they were severely shamed for making mistakes or getting it wrong in the eyes of the authority. This may have been combined with little understanding of their particular struggles or little attempt to help them remedy or learn from mistakes. In many ways this shame-based educational process feeds into the driver behaviour outlined above and mitigates against any true learning or creativity and spontaneity of expression.

One of our first principles is that there are no absolute 'right' interventions but only more or less effective interventions depending on the outcome you desire. Often the idea of doing it right has got caught up in morality as though it is immoral to make a mistake! We stress that making a mistake is part of the learning process! Striving to behave within your own moral code and with integrity may nevertheless mean making mistakes and learning from these!

Case example

How might you manage the following situation?

You are supervisor in a small tutor group of three people. To date you have had about four meetings with the tutor group. You think that Jill and Jack have taken to supervision well and use it effectively to learn and reflect on the group programme. Joanna, on the other hand, seems to drain the energy of the group. At every opportunity she talks about herself, her past, the difficult times at home. She relates this to almost all the situations brought to supervision and what she brings herself is related and explored by her in a similar ego-centred way. What can you do as supervisor?

Review and discussion

1. Have you a sense of the stages that supervisees go through on their journey to becoming more skilled in their profession?
2. Where are you on this journey and what are the tasks and challenges you face just now?
3. What are the skills you bring to your work just now?
4. Can you see how transference might work within supervision?
5. Have you worked out what 'drivers' you have developed?

Supervisee Skills

The following seven chapters present seven key skills on which being an effective supervisee are based. In our experience, the more you are able to practice these skills, the more you will be able to use supervision as a highly effective learning relationship.

The seven skills are:

1. Learning how to learn.
2. Learning from experience.
3. Learning how to reflect.
4. Learning how to give and receive feedback.
5. Learning realistic self-evaluation.
6. Learning emotional awareness.
7. Learning how to dialogue.

We will look in some detail at each of these key skills in turn…

CHAPTER 8

Supervisee Skill No. 1: Learning How to Learn

Throughout this book we have insisted that supervision is to encourage and support the learning of supervisees. This section is to help you, the supervisee understand what learning is and to identify your particular style of learning. Individuals have their preferred ways of learning and learn at different paces. We also know that learning is influenced by social interaction, interpersonal relationship and communications with others, by past experiences of learning and past learning relationships. Some people learn primarily by doing, others by reflecting, others by theorising and again, others who are pragmatists and love to learn by applying theory to practice (see Appendix 8 for a description of Honey and Mumford's [1992] Learning Styles and where to access their Learning Styles Inventory).

Our question for you is…

How do you learn?

We are making a distinction between teaching and learning. In teaching, the teacher asks you to join him/her in their world. In learning, the teacher joins you in your world. Effective supervisors are flexible and move towards the supervisee. They see it as their task to find out how supervisees learn and then adapt their teaching strategies to facilitate learning. Supervisors can only do this when they know the individualised learning format of their supervisee. Some supervisors use a 'one-size-fits-all' concept of learning, i.e., that all supervisees learn in the same way. We think this is unfortunate and results in forcing some supervisees to learn in ways that are not appropriate for them.

Exercise

1. What has been the most significant learning in your life in the past five years? Why?
2. Who has been the most significant person in your learning? Why?
3. If you could learn something that would make a huge difference in your life just now, what is it? Why don't you learn it?

The point of this exercise is to help you begin to think of how you learn, what kinds of people facilitate your learning and what blocks your learning. Look in particular at your answers to the questions *why* and *why don't you learn*?

What is learning?

Have a look at some definitions and make some notes of what they mean to you in the light of the exercise above.

1. *'Learning is what you do when you don't know what to do'* (Claxton, 1999).
2. *'Learning is the changes a person makes in himself or herself that increase the know-why and/or the know-what and/or the know-how the person possesses in respect of a given subject'* (Vaill, 1996, p. 21).

Adult learning

What are the principles of adult learning? As an adult learner, you will be asked to take responsibility for implementing some of these principles:

Principles:

1. Adults learn best when they take responsibility for their own learning, i.e., they have an internal motivation to learn.
2. Adult learning depends on adults being involved in planning, implementing and evaluating their own learning.
3. Self-direction is important for adult learning.
4. Adults learn best when they are in touch with their own particular way of learning (auditory, visual, kinesthetic).
5. Emotions are as much a part of learning as is intellect for adults.
6. Adults respond, like all learners, to a facilitative learning environment and good learning relationships.
7. Adults respond particularly well to experiential learning.
8. Language is a key part of learning.

You can probably add other factors to these principles that affect and help your learning (challenge, feedback, support, groups, reading, etc.).

There are many forms of learning:

1. Knowledge, information, models, theories and frameworks. This is usually intellectual knowledge.
2. Skills that allow us to do more, relate better, solve problems, work in teams, etc.

3. Accessing intelligences other than our preferred one (Gardner, 1999; Goleman, 1996, 1998; Zohar & Marshall, 2001) increases our learning and our learning about learning.

4. Knowing our learning style and the learning styles of others can assist as we set up learning experiences for ourselves and others (Honey & Mumford, 1992).

5. Transformational learning investigates the assumptions and beliefs we bring to our learning. In looking at the underlying structure of our ways of knowing (of how we make sense of our world) we come to know, and begin to question, whether these assumptions and beliefs curtail or advance our learning.

6. Experiential learning allows us insight from an action/reflection stance. We do, reflect on our doing, learn from our reflection, and apply new learning to our tasks.

7. Internal learning pulls us within to look at our values, our way of being, our self-awareness. In going within, we learn how to manage ourselves, how to build personal qualities for our lives, how to liberate potential and, in particular, learn how to learn.

8. Tacit learning is that store of learning we have without sometimes realising we have it—ways of doing things without knowing how or why.

9. Intuition—a non-rational way of knowing that allows us to come to decisions and find ways of doing things without going through the rational process.

From the above we suggest three levels of learning:

1. **Level 1:** The *what* of learning: information, theories, frameworks, skills.

2. **Level 2:** The *how* of learning: understanding how you learn in your own particular way.

3. **Level 3:** The *why* of learning: discovering why you learn the way you do.

The following table outlines various aspects of these ways of learning:

	Strength	Limitation	Methods	Result
Level 1 (What)	Problem Solving Information Skills	Nothing Changes Head Knowledge Incongruence Never Question	Lecturing Reading Theories Frameworks Skills Training	Knowledge Skills
Level 2 (How)	Know My Style I Own My Learning Use Variety	Individualistic Reject Knowledge Only One Voice	Experiential Learning Lifelong Learning Feedback Reflection	Personal Insight Emotions
Level 3 (Why)	Ongoing Change Process	Individualistic No Real World Subjectivity	Dialogue Questioning Reflection Dilemmas	Transforming Questioning

Table 1: The Aspects of the Three Levels of Learning

Using Table 1, begin to think of what level of learning comes easily to you and which levels are difficult.

Different forms of intelligences

Gardner (1999) has suggested there are different intelligences—not just the intellectual. We have added another one: spiritual intelligence, from Zohar and Marshall (2001). Have a look at these and see which intelligence seems closest to where you are.

Gardner's seven intelligences

1. **Linguistic:** Language, writing, storytelling and poetry. Sensitivity to words and their sounds: puns and poems. Learn through listening, writing, reading and discussing. Predominantly auditory system.

2. **Mathematical and logical:** Problem solvers who delight in sequence and order and logic. Deductive and inductive reasoning. They are good at solving puzzles and abstract thinking, see the pattern in things. They are good also at hard data, evidence, assessments and hypotheses. Seek harmony and order.

3. **Visual and spatial:** Ability to see things from different angles. Ability to visualise and imagine scenes. Imagination. Learns through models and diagrams.

4. **Musical:** Discerns patterns in sound and enjoys experimenting with them. Shows sensitivity to mood changes and picks out individual sounds. Aware of changes within themselves from music, good sense of rhythm. Will enjoy singing.

5. **Interpersonal:** Learns by entering and making sense of the world of others. Learns from group experiences and collaborative learning. Good at social relationships and learns from them. Good at influencing and listening.

6. **Intrapersonal:** Knowledge about self—can access one's own moods and feelings. Learns from inner world and seeks explanations from within. Values personal growth, enjoys reflective times.

7. **Kinesthetic:** Uses the body in learning ways—artists, dancers, actors, machinists, and jewellers. Skill in the muscle. Learns from touch, movement, manipulation and physical experience. Will enjoy doing—field trips etc..

and…

8. **Spiritual:** *'The intelligence with which we address and solve problems of meaning and value, the intelligence with which we can place our actions and our lives in a wider, meaning-giving context, the intelligence with which we can assess that one course of action or one life-path is more meaningful than another.'* (Zohar & Marshall, 2000).

Levels of learning

Hawkins and Smith (2006) connect four focus points of learning to interventions. These four can also form the basis of different supervision conversations. The four are:

1. **Skills or competencies** (they define a competency as the ability to utilise a skill or use a tool): By and large a skill is the ability to do something well. People such as managers, friends, parents can set up skills training which is taught usually through instruction. In supervision you will learn a number of skills: how to contract with your clients, how to intervene successfully,

how to make ethical decisions and how to deal with critical moments in the relationship.

2. **Performance and capability** (a capability is the ability to use a skill at the right time, in the right way and in the right place): moves away somewhat from skills (inputs) to helping individuals advance more in their jobs. It could add to skills in helping an individual be more assertive, or manage conflict in their team or be more proactive in dealing with colleagues. With performance focus the individual needs to be connected to skills and behaviours that make an increase in their ability to do their job well. Instruction, coaching and training would be the normal interventions used here.

3. **Developmental learning:** is somewhat longer term and helps individuals think and act more holistically: as a person, as a professional. It is wider in its focus and could help a manager prepare for a more responsible role in the organisation. Coaching and mentoring would be the educational process involved at this stage. Hawkins and Smith (2006) might call this a capacity (a human quality such as flexibility, warmth, etc.).

4. **Transformational learning:** enables individuals to shift gear into another way of perceiving. Part of the process in transformational learning is the evaluation of old mindsets and mental maps. With transformational learning comes new ways of perceiving and looking at situations. It thinks more systemically and allows individuals to connect more to the bigger picture. Hawkins and Smith (2006) call *developmental learning* a 'capacity in level' and see *transformational* learning as capacity between levels.

Exercise

Appendices 8 and 9 are two outlines to help you focus on your learning style and will help you discern which intelligence seems more suited to you. Stop here and do both.

Personalised learning

More awareness of experiential learning along with both social role models of supervision and developmental models of supervision meant that supervisors became facilitators, providers or managers of experiential learning rather than teachers (Carroll, 1996; Holloway, 1995). There was a movement away from teaching to learning, and a clear understanding that these two were not necessarily connected in supervision. Research by Tannenbaum (1997) supports this movement and unearths the surprisingly low percentage of learning attributed to formal learning programmes. Supervision now joins other professional learning interventions such as coaching and mentoring as being a form of 'personalised' or 'customised' learning. There is a clear emphasis on the learning style, learning intelligence and individualised learning formats of the supervisee. Supervisors, not supervisees, are the ones who accommodate, who move, become flexible and adapt their supervisory interventions to meet the learning styles of supervisees. Peter Hawkins uses a telling phase to make this point: *'If you are saying the same things to more than one of your supervisees, the chances are you are supervising yourself'* (Keynote Address, BASPR Conference, July 2007).

Exercise

In the light of your knowledge and insights from the previous exercise, imagine that I will be your supervisor. Can you answer some questions for me?
1. What is your learning style?
2. How can I best facilitate your learning?
3. What can I do that helps you learn best?
4. What blocks your learning?
5. What might I do that would block your learning?

Exercise

Have a look at the teaching strategies in Appendix 12 and see, as you go through them, which ones seem to suit your style of learning best. Can you share these with your supervisor so that he/she has some insights into how best to facilitate your learning?

Conclusion

Our hope is that, at this stage, you have some good insights into your particular style and method of learning and can begin to negotiate with your supervisor about how he/she can facilitate that learning.

Case example

John is one of the supervisees in your group of three. He is quite experienced as a Tutor and has already run this particular programme many times. You can see he finds it difficult to take on the supervisee role and is constantly edging towards being the co-leader with you as supervisor in the group. You sense that he doesn't really think he needs supervision and that he feels he is far more experienced and able than the other members of the supervision group. He has specialised in psychoanalytic theory and is constantly reminding the group, who do not know too much about it, how valuable it is and how applicable to the situations brought to supervision. You feel deskilled and somewhat put down especially since last week when he expressed surprise you had not read a current book. You are preparing to give him some feedback on how he is presenting himself in supervision.

Review and discussion

1. Can you begin to describe what learning styles exist and what different types of learning take place?
2. Could you now outline for me your style of learning?
3. If I was your supervisor, how best could I facilitate your learning in supervision?
4. What are the main challenges for you as a learner?

CHAPTER 9

Supervisee Skill No. 2: Learning from Experience

Supervision is the forum we set up to learn from our work, and our practice is the focus of supervision. Reflecting on practice in order to learn from it is what makes supervision supervision. No practice, no supervision. We stop doing and begin a reflective, collaborative dialogue around the experiences we have been through. With another, or others, or on our own, we sit at the feet of our experience; we allow our experience to become our teacher. We present our experience and listen as others help us observe and tell stories about that experience. We learn primarily in supervision not from books, or even the supervisor, or the gurus, or the theories, but from experience itself. Supervision is a form of learning from experience.

In supervision:

1. data becomes information;
2. information becomes knowledge;
3. knowledge becomes wisdom;
4. wisdom becomes practical action.

Experience has to be shifted, examined, analysed, considered and interpreted in order to move it to knowledge, wisdom and action—that is the role of supervision.

How does this happen and how do supervisees learn the skill of making meaning from their experience? What process do we go through in order to learn from our own experience and how can supervision facilitate that process?

Experiential learning and learning from experience

We want to make an unusual distinction here in order to understand how experience teaches us: there is *experiential learning* and *learning from experience* and we suggest they are not the same. Learning from experience is where we deliberately and consciously set out to learn from what happens to us, whereas experiential learning is where our experience teaches us unconsciously, without our setting out to learn from it. A cat learns fast—who will feed it, where food can be found, what is helpful for it and unhelpful. A baby does too—it knows very soon that putting its hand on a hot stove is very painful and it learns quickly and permanently not to do that again. The baby or the cat didn't set out to learn about hot stoves, or how to walk, or what food tastes good—these learnings come from the experience, unconsciously and implicitly outside of our awareness. Learning from experience, on the other hand, is a specifically human endeavour where we hold experience up to the light and begin to work with it in order to learn from it. In supervision, the method by which we do that learning is reflection: we stop, we think, we feel and then comes the insight—*"I can see why I reacted so strongly to that client, he is just like my brother"*. The sequence of what happens in this process is as follows: *data*—e.g., the strong feeling of competition I had with the client—is *reflected on* (Why did I feel that way? I am curious I reacted in a way I don't usually react), and becomes *knowledge*—e.g., he reminds me of my brother and he and I were always competing—which in turn allows me choice in what I will do, e.g., he is not my brother, I don't need to compete with him, and I will watch to ensure competition doesn't happen in our sessions together. Reflection becomes the difference between learning from experience (I begin a process of deliberation) and experiential learning (where I learn without reflection).

It is not automatic

It might seem strange to say, but we are not always good learners from our own experience—learning from experience does not happen automatically. The price we pay for not learning from experience is that we tend to repeat what has happened rather than have other choices. Note the following example: *'Not long ago a medical study showed that if heart doctors tell their seriously at-risk patients they will literally die if they do not make changes to their personal lives—diet, exercise, smoking—still only one in seven is actually able to change. One in seven. And we can safely assume that the other six wanted to live, see more sunsets, watch their grandchildren grow up. They didn't lack a sense of urgency. The incentives for change could not be greater. The doctors made sure they knew just what they needed to do. Still, they couldn't do it'* (Kegan & Lahey, 2009, p. 1). This is a good example of people not being able to learn from experience what is good for them, even when they face a life or death situation. One of the seven presumably learned by allowing the experience to impact them sufficiently, reflected on it deeply enough and organised their lives to exclude what is unhealthy for them.

Learning from experience or learning from the experience of others

Our first question is, do we look to our own experience or the experience of others as the primary guide for knowledge? We start with our own experience. Well, actually, most of us don't. There is a tendency to start with the experience of others and use it as a norm and guide for life and work. *This is knowing from outside ourselves.* The process of socialisation usually demands that we adopt the learnings of others as guidelines for our lives before we begin the often painful practice of choosing our own values and ways of living. *This is knowing from inside ourselves.* The underlying process, often unarticulated, is: trust in the knowledge and wisdom of others, adopt their values and ways of making meaning, live from within their experience rather than your own. The more liberal among us might add: before you begin to use your own experience as a guide to your life. The less liberal amongst us might say: don't trust your own experience at all, it lets you down; there are wiser, more expert, more knowledgeable people out there who know what is good or better for you than you do. So for many people, the journey to using their own experience as a springboard for learning doesn't happen, and they continue to let the experience of others be the norm for interpreting their own experience. Rarely do we change the process around and suggest that primary experience is the best teacher, learn to trust it, learn how to reflect on it, and learn how to make it our primary source of knowledge and truth.

We start with the experience of others and sift and make sense of our own experience through their experience. We are strong imitation learners. Books are valuable sources of knowledge, information and wisdom, but unless you have written the book yourself, it contains the experience/s of another or others. You may adopt or adapt its contents to your own life and allow its guidelines and principles to direct and influence how you live. The works of Freud and Jung are examples, as are The Bible or the Koran. They are narratives outlining the experiences of individuals and a group of people and show how those individuals and groups made sense of their lives and how they give meaning to human behaviour. Many people take these texts as a guide and mediate their own lives and experiences through them. They make sense of their lives and sift and filter their experiences through an interpreter. That interpreter can be wisdom traditions (religions, cults, philosophies, theories, handed-on guidelines) that play a similar role in people's lives and covertly and often overtly suggest they take prime place in helping individuals, groups and organisations name their values and direct their actions. We can list lots of other areas in the *'experience by proxy'* (Gelb, 1999) approach to what we accept as helpful in making meaning of our lives—television, mentors, parents, teachers, etc. All start with the belief that it's best to start with the experience, learning and wisdom of others in the choices and values we adopt in life.

First, we suggest the person stays with their own experience and uses it as the springboard for their learning, turning to the experience of others second as a comparison and support to their own learning from experience. How often is our experience speaking to us, calling to us, shouting at us, screaming at us—when will we heed it, listen, make sense of it and allow it to lead us to transformational learning? Poor old personal experience—it wants to be heard.

On the continuum of *'trust the experience of others absolutely'* to the further end of *'trust only my own experience'* there are lots of positions where at times we trust our experience, at other times we go with the wisdom and guidance and experience of others through to various blends of those two. You can read further on these positions in Strenger (2005) and Coupland (1991).

It seems to us that we don't trust our own experience enough. Even when our own experience is shouting at us, we listen to the experience of others first. One of us was running a conference day in Dublin. There were about 150 people in the room. One man, after the first experiential exercise, took the microphone and made a criticism of the environment: *"I couldn't hear myself speak, the room was too noisy, there were too many people in the room—it ruined the exercise for me."* The reply was, *"So why didn't you and your small group leave and find a quiet place?"* His reply was, *"Could we have done that? I didn't know we had permission"*. How interesting—he read his experience, knew what it was saying to him but didn't act on it because he made a series of assumptions. If he had stopped and allowed himself to be disoriented, concluded that this was not working for him and reflected on his options, he could have decided on another pathway.

One man who arguably deserves the title, *'the patron saint of learning from experience'*, is Leonardo da Vinci. He is a strong contender as the champion of the value of personal experience as our best teacher: *'...throughout his life he proudly referred to himself as* unomo senza lettere *(man without letters) and* discepolo della esperiencza *(disciple of experience)'* (Gelb, 1999). Da Vinci wrote, *'To me it seems that those sciences are vain and full of error which are not born of experience, mother of all certainty, firsthand experience which in its origins, or means, or end has passed through one of the five senses'* (Gelb, 1999, p. 78). A fierce commitment to firsthand knowledge, he questioned authority, certainty and imitation.

However, and this is where he is a true integrationist, he also read widely, consulted others and their works, and kept a large library—he was certainly not averse to accessing the experience of others. But these 'experiences by proxy', which is what he called the thoughts and ideas of others, were tested ultimately in the fire of his own experience. He raised experience to the greatest of learning heights: *'Experience never errs: it is only your judgement that errs in promising itself results as are not caused by your experience'* (Gelb, 1999, p. 79). How you interpret, make sense of and give meaning to your experience is open to question, not the experience itself.

The process of learning from experience

A key issue in learning from experience is how we make meaning of the events in our lives. We are meaning making animals, i.e., we attribute meaning to what happens to us. We either do that in the way we have always learned: through myths (e.g., don't trust someone whose eyebrows meet); through stereotypes (e.g., all Italians love food, Afro-Caribbeans just want to play music and not work, etc.); or defence mechanisms (e.g., it's never my fault; you are giving me feedback because you don't like me); or we find some new way of making meaning. When information hits us our first port of call is to interpret it according to our past ways of interpreting information. We already have moulds into which we try to fit new information and make sense and meaning of it in a traditional way.

Or we find another way to make meaning of it. We don't confine ourselves to a single interpretation but instead know there are many, and we allow ourselves to sift through the myriad possibilities. The fact that my client has not appeared for our counselling or coaching session can have many possible meanings. If I stick with one (e.g., he doesn't really want to be here and his absence is a message telling me this) I could be right, but not having considered the other possibilities means I haven't accessed what the meaning might be from the perspective of the client.

There is a fascinating book written just to make this point. Raymond Queneau, a French author, first published this book in 1947 entitled, *'Exercises in Style'*. Queneau tells a very simple half page story and then retells it in 124 different ways, styles, and meanings. The point he makes is that any event, any happening, can be *proliferated almost to infinity'* and can be interpreted in an amazing number of ways—there is a *'dynamic fluidity of lived experience'* (Knibb, 2010) and an *'infinite possibility of meaning'* (Derrida, 1981)—there are innumerable ways to tell it. An event that has no point anyway can be interpreted in a multitude of ways depending on a number of factors: what you saw and heard; what you allowed yourself to see and hear; the background you come from; how you made sense of this in the past; your culture, language, etc. Supervision and learning from experience builds on the premise that what happens to us in our work has many ways of being interpreted, and supervision is our time for looking at some of these.

So supervision is a forum where we retell the stories and events of our practice and begin the journey of making sense of them. We tell our supervisory story from within our own understanding and then we try to get outside our own understanding to look at the ways others might interpret that event. I tell you *my* story in supervision, and then I listen as you tell me *your* story about my story from outside my story. You could think of supervision as a series of lenses through which you look with zoom in and zoom out (wide lens, narrow lens). We tell the story, we retell from other angles and perspectives and points of view and styles. In the retelling we see and hear and understand more and more, and we go back to our work with more wisdom, insight and better understanding. Though Queneau never uses the term, his book is about different ways of making meaning.

So back to our question. How do we use supervision to learn from our experience of the work we do? The framework (illustrated in Figure 2) looks complicated, but stay with us as we go through it. It incorporates Left-hand Column Learning (illustrated in Figures 3–9 that follow), and Right-hand Column Learning (illustrated in Figures 10–14 that follow). We think it is a good way to set up your experience deliberately so that you learn from it.

Left-hand Column Learning

Right-hand Column Learning

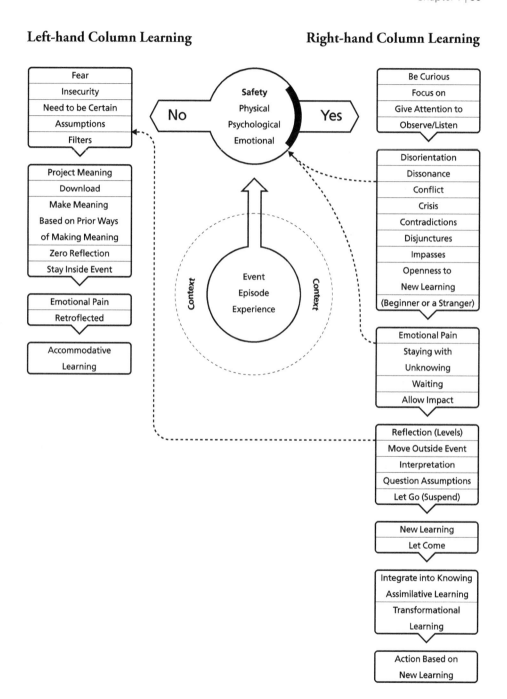

Figure 2: The Process of Learning from Experience

Some of the processes involved

In learning from experience we move from evaluation to curiosity. Instead of going into evaluation (e.g., How stupid I am to put my hand on a hot stove, or I really got the way I challenged that client wrong), I entice or invoke curiosity (e.g., Why did I do that? What was happening in my life that distracted me? I wonder if I am unconsciously punishing myself?) Can we start with curiosity and then move to evaluation, not the other way around. An excellent supervision question is, *'Can you tell it to me again from a curious perspective?'*

An Event Happens

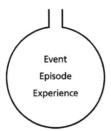

Figure 3: An Event Happens

All happenings can be events which are a once-off (e.g., Gary challenged his client in what he thought was an appropriate way and the client reacted very negatively and told him he felt dismissed); episodes which are a series of events over a short period of time (e.g., there is a person in your group who remains remote and uninvolved over time despite your best efforts to bring him in); and/or experiences which can last a long time (over the year you have been counselling someone but they still continue to ask that you rescue them and give them the answers they need). In the three examples you are puzzled, not sure what is happening, trying to make sense of the interactions and relationships and wondering what is the best way ahead.

Like every experience each of these three happen in a context.

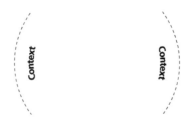

Figure 4: Every Experience Happens in a Context

Bateson (2000) used to say, *'The context gives meaning'*. The context is vitally important in so far as it often automatically provides inherited meaning. The context of Michael growing up as a catholic in Belfast or Maria growing up white in apartheid South Africa meant inheriting a whole set of filters, assumptions, expectations, directives, loyalties, etc., all of which provided a pre-determined meaning. The context of the organisation in which I work, the context of the culture in which I am embedded, all contribute to how I make sense of my experiences. All these automatically bring sets of meanings already established. Until I question that meaning it often remains the sole way in which I can make sense of experiences that happen to me. It was a 'given' in the sense that I 'clicked into' the experience of others and allowed their experience to direct and give meaning to my experience. One of our supervisees is an organisational consultant who is coaching an executive. She is telling me about the strong reactions and feelings she has during her coaching session. I ask her if she has shared these with the coachee. She would normally but she hasn't. As we unravel the issue we realise she too has been silenced, like the coachee and like many others in this company. The context demands silence.

Left-hand column learning

The next reaction is quite important. There will be an emotional reaction on my part to the event, the episode, or the experience, and that emotional reaction will have its basis in safety. How safe am I? If unsafe and insecure, I may well head for *Accommodative Learning* (or what we call *Left-hand Column Learning*) where I project my meaning onto the event from pre-existing knowledge, information or learnings. So in the episode with Gary above, when Gary is not emotionally safe in supervision, he might not share what happened with his supervisor. He might evaluate immediately and conclude he got it wrong. In the example of the organisational consultant above, the consultant was not curious but evaluative: *"I am making a mess of this, this client is resistant—she is projecting old meanings"*.

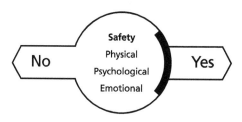

Figure 5: Safety

This is where safety becomes so important. I won't question or become curious, but remain evaluative, until I am safe, sometimes physically, but certainly emotionally and psychologically. There are two types of safety here. The first is the desperate need for safety that doesn't allow me to think or experiment or try out or risk, or question. This safety keeps me where I am. The result is that many people have limited choice in their making meaning from their experience (learning from their experience) other than the learnings they have been provided with and which have been handed on to them. This sends them down the left-hand side of Figure 2. Fear is activated which, in turn, connects us to the Reptilian Brain. Now we are dealing with a desperate quest for safety, using fight, flight, fragment or freeze as our strategies, and basically have one way or very limited ways to make sense of what is happening. Often we will see ourselves as victims. Left-hand column learning is often a way to avoid learning.

Angela Brew (1993) uses herself as an example of avoiding learning by using learning itself:

'I did not want to know and I feared even facing the fact that I did not want to know. I have a whole repertoire of mechanisms and procedures to prevent me from finding out what I don't want to know. What is acceptable and unacceptable knowledge? The learning we do can be a way of avoiding what we need to know or should know. Our whole lives can be a defence against knowing those things we least want to acknowledge. We can build a whole edifice of knowledge in order to avoid facing what we do not want to know.'

The figure below summarises some of the backgrounds that keep us from learning from our experience.

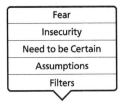

Figure 6: Backgrounds that Keep us from Learning

What affects our learning from experience (makes us learn from experience in narrow, congested ways)? If I am afraid, if I am not secure and safe, then I will begin to project meaning onto the event or the experience. This client is resistant and doesn't want to be here. It is hard for me at times to get outside and become an observer of my own experiences. We become so caught into the experiences themselves that we cannot see them from some distance. They envelop us. There are a number of barriers to learning from experience each of which limits us in our way of making sense of what is happening. Often we will see ourselves as victims. It will also release what the Transactional Analysis people refer to as: *'script'*, *'adaptation'*, *'discounting'* and *'elements of attachment'* that are well-formed. All these will offer predetermined ways to make sense of experience (embedded filters and assumptions in our lives) that often do not allow us to entertain other possible interpretations (e.g., *"I was always told I couldn't sing"*—I adopt the script and live it out. I never allow myself to think it could be otherwise). I may be so caught in these scripts emotionally that I cannot see them from a distance. The result will be accommodative learning that accommodates or integrates the new event into old learning. Nothing changes as a result and the new event is confirmed as affirmation of existing ways of knowing. The result is projected meaning (or downloading) and imprisons new experiences in old meanings.

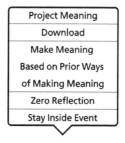

Figure 7: Meanings

Emotional pain may be retroflected (turned in on oneself) or projected out. I might begin to see myself as the victim here (retroflected pain) or look to you as the enemy and the problem (projected meaning).

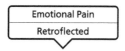

Figure 8: Emotional Pain

One of us was working as a coach with a man whose experience was shouting at him to leave the toxic environment of his job, but he was too frightened and fearful to allow himself to consider that option. The pain of this was brought inside himself (he became depressed) and, at times, was projected out in a view of how terrible the organisation was because it did not understand him (even though he had never tried to explain his situation to them).

```
┌─────────────────────┐
│   Accommodative     │
│     Learning        │
└─────────────────────┘
```

Figure 9: Accommodative Learning

The end result of Left-hand Column Learning is Accommodative Learning.

As human beings, we make meaning of our situations and we do it in an instant. What is the process by which we make meaning? The first thing we do in making meaning is to unconsciously filter the data of our surroundings, and test it against pre-established expectations and assumptions, e.g., like the man in the conference hall in Ireland who attached his own meaning to the event presumably in the light of former experience. He assumed there was no permission to leave the room, that the expectation was that people remain where they were for the duration of the exercise no matter how unhelpful the environment. He trusted my experience, rather than his own.

Right-hand column learning

Learning from experience is an interpretative process. Experiences are just events: it is how we experience them and how we use them that turns them into learning and hopefully wisdom—it is in dialogue with our experiences that experiential learning is turned into propositional learning. Critical reflection is required to expose the taken-for-granted assumptions we make. Socialisation constructs us, reflection deconstructs and reconstructs us.

When something happens and I am safe enough to take the risk I can allow myself to hold the space of listening, or focusing on, of being curious about. Allowing this into my consciousness will, of course, throw me. One supervisee said, *"It's not working, it should work, the theory is there—tell me what I am doing wrong?"*. When the reply was, *"Maybe it doesn't work here—let's see if your experience can help you find another way"*, it placed the supervisee at a crossroads. Do I keep doing what I should be doing, have been told or should I stop and think, trust my experience and learn another way?

Moving down the right-hand side of the diagram involves us in a learning that is different to accommodative learning. While the context pulls us to make sense of experiences in former ways, when we are safe physically, emotionally and mentally enough we can begin to allow ourselves to be curious. The thick black line in Figure 2 (and replicated in Figure 5) illustrates the barrier that exists in beginning this journey. Sometimes it is difficult to allow ourselves to question, to notice, to give attention to, to observe the very things that might be against our previous ways of knowing, our knowledge and our loyalties.

What would it be like if a Catholic in Northern Ireland allowed himself or herself to look at Protestant neighbours, be curious about who they are and why they think the way they do, be open to new ways of making sense of their behaviour (rather than the old way I have inherited). Scharmer (2007) puts it well: *'The first part of this process is to observe, observe, observe, which means stop the downloading and open up into a full immersion into the context. Then you retreat and reflect, allowing the inner knowing to emerge. You access your own source. So you go from the chaos of observation to the still, inner place where knowing comes to the surface…It requires a letting go of your old self in order to find your emerging authentic self.'*

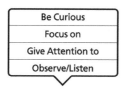

Figure 10: Access Your own Source

At all stages there is a temptation to pull back to old ways of thinking. The pull becomes stronger as I get into areas of unknowing, of emotional pain, of dissonance, especially if I am asked to give up ways of thinking that have sustained me for a long time. There may also be loyalties involved—to communities, to religious or political schools of thought. Allowing right-hand column thinking can put me in conflict with other ways of thinking. Rumi said: *"In the field beyond right and wrong, I will meet you there"*. This could be a mantra for transformational learning. Not only does it take courage at times to continue down the Right-hand Column Learning, but it also demands compassion and support for oneself and others.

The first part of the right-hand column learning process involves use of the Limbic system (limbic resonance and regulation) as we stay in touch with what is happening, trust the experience, and wait at times when there is no clear way forward. We read inner worlds—our own and others—and we stay with our sensation and awareness. This time has all the feelings of transition time—caught between knowing and not knowing, having let go and when 'letting come' has not yet happened. How we feel is illustrated in Figure 11.

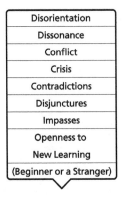

Disorientation
Dissonance
Conflict
Crisis
Contradictions
Disjunctures
Impasses
Openness to
New Learning
(Beginner or a Stranger)

Figure 11: We Feel

The second part of the right-hand column learning process is where the Frontal Cortex (Executive or Human Brain) is activated and we now move into reflection and new meanings (interpretations). We allow ourselves to reflect openly, honestly, with integrity and authenticity. We go with where the experience is taking us (gay and lesbian sexuality is another way of expressing sexuality; these people are not my enemies, they are afraid like me; my avowed counselling orientation is limited in dealing with this problem; I realise how judgemental I am about certain groups of people).

Some of the features of this time are:

1. The period of time involved can be short or long. Some people take years to make a decision they have been struggling with (ending a relationship, coming to terms with a loss, choosing a career they want rather than one that is chosen for them) and go through a lot of emotional pain as they search for what this means and how they can learn from it in order to make a decision (a 'faithful action') that is true to who they are.

2. Right-hand Column Learning is about the ability to move outside the experience and begin to see it from other perspectives. In Left-hand Column Learning there is an immersion in the experience itself that

does not allow us to have distance from it (particularly emotional and psychological distance).

3. Right-hand Column Learning almost always involves loss and giving up and letting go (what Zuboff & Maxim, 2002 call *'committing little murders'*)—it sometimes involves us in conflicts and disagreements with others, especially those who have shared my way of making meaning of events.

4. It also goes through a process of introjection, integration and internalisation until the transformational learning becomes part of who I am.

5. This type of learning involves courage, compassion and conflict and is often a journey of undoing past learnings and unmaking past decisions.

When something happens and I am safe enough to take the risk, I can allow myself to hold a space for listening, focusing and curiosity. Allowing this into my consciousness will, of course, throw me. On the other hand, when I allow myself (intentionally or unconsciously) to be thrown by the event I can be open to learning from my emotional response, as outlined in Figure 12.

Emotional Pain	Limbic System (Reading the Internal Worlds of Self and Others)
Impasse (Stuck)	Am I Safe?
Either... or Choice,	Can I Embrace My Hypocrisies?
Confusion	Can I Face Fear?
Waiting	Can I Move from Hiding?
Allow the Impact	Can I Allow Myself to be Vulnerable?

Figure 12: Emotional Response

With disorientation and confusion, it is not easy to stay with what is happening. In this type of learning we need to allow the impact of what is happening to hit us. We stay with the impact. When we move too quickly into evaluation or acceptance/rejection we move from the learning. Sometimes *not* thinking about what is happening is helpful. Let the unspoken, the unsaid, even inarticulate, event be with you. Allow what is evoked or elicited by the event to come. This is the part where we plunge into reality and immerse ourselves in the experience. The challenge at this point is to stay authentic and remain resilient. It is also a time to be 'indifferent' (not unconcerned, but not prematurely concluding; passionate about what is happening, but not already at the destination—in fact I am prepared to go to the destination that emerges). We live in an unpredictable world, as described by Jarvis (2008): '... *in novel situations throughout life we have new sensations, so that we can rarely take the world for granted: we enter a state of disjuncture and implicitly we raise questions: What do I do now? What does this mean? What is that smell? The sound? And so on—there is a sense of unknowing'* (p. 19). Often the place of ignorance and unknowing is the point of transformation. I allow myself to be unsure, not to know, to stay with confusion in my sea of unknowing. I sharpen my attention.

All sorts of resistances at this stage begin to emerge: our commitment to making the time available; the painfulness of the experience; being defended; strong feelings; blaming; and so on, can bubble to the surface and tempt us to retreat to a place of no new learning. There is sometimes conflict with others, sometimes my closest others, my community. We need to be self-aware, to know ourselves, to know our characteristic way to avoid and deny, and to know the pitfalls that would stop us from staying true to new learning. We resist having our world dismantled. It can be valuable at this stage to talk or write about what is happening, to 'get it out', and to allow others to see and comment. Sometimes we have to face up to the negatives within, our guilt and shame. We enter the world of reflection: we see from where we are, from the position and stance we have taken in life. Can I take another viewpoint, enter another world and see the event from within that world? It is different when you participate rather than remain an observer. We bring mind sets, beliefs, mental maps and assumptions to what we see, hear, touch, feel and smell. These are often unexamined and untested for their friendliness.

But now, I go into a place of unknowing where I need to suspend my knowing for a while. This is often a difficult place as I wait and stay with the unknowing. We let go of our knowing, our filters, our certainty, our sureness and we stay with the unknown.

We move to reflection and learning. This is a movement into the Executive Brain (Frontal Cortex part of the brain) where we begin to click into the rational and the problem-solving capability we have while not forgetting to stay with the limbic and the emotional. We have included the six levels of reflection in the middle box here (even though they are not in Figure 2). We will present and discuss the six levels in the next chapter.

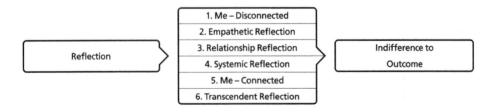

Figure 13: Rational Problem Solving

Through reflection and reflexivity (the person doing the reflection) I will now see how I reflect and how I make meaning of events. I will be challenged to let go of my control, my insecurity, my greed, etc., and think in bigger and wider pictures.

Don't underestimate the pain and losses at this stage of learning. You may need moral support to help you move through these stages.

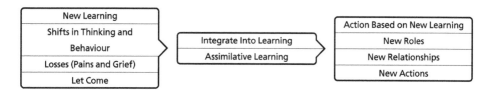

Figure 14: The Need for Moral Support

Conclusion

One of the greatest gifts we have as humans is our ability to use our experience to learn—where we give attention deliberately and intentionally to what has happened to us, or is happening to us, as a method of learning from that experience. As we say in this chapter, that process can go either way. The first is towards *accommodative learning* where the experience is accommodated according to old ways of learning. The second way is towards *transformative learning*—where we allow the new experience to transform our ways of thinking that result in new learning and therefore new behaviour. Supervision is one of the best environments for doing this.

Example

Della has been disoriented and clearly thrown by what has happened. In the last session with her client, at a tense and difficult moment, she wondered out loud if the client knew what the connections were between what was happening at her work and herself. The client quietly said, "Yes, I was abused as a child and withdrew behind a veil of silence and tears". Della waited with her. About 10 minutes later, her client looked up and with anger shouted, "How could you do this to me? You don't understand. This is cruel". The client then walked out even though they had 20 minutes left of their session. Della immediately goes into evaluation and defence mode. She evaluates herself as unhelpful and unskilled, and evaluates her client as not being able to deal with what has happened in her life. How might you help Della with Right-hand Column Learning?

Review and discuss

1. What do you think is your characteristic way of making meaning from experience?

2. Take an event (an event, an episode or an experience) in your life (personal life or work life) and see if you can make meaning of it using the framework above?

3. How might you prepare for supervision using the Process of Learning from the Experience framework above?

CHAPTER 10

Supervisee Skill No.3: Learning How to Reflect

'The moment one gives close attention to anything, even a blade of grass, it becomes a mysterious, awesome, indescribably magnificent world in itself' (Henry Miller).

'The man approached the sage and said, "Oh, Master, I have travelled far and wide to hear the three secrets that I need to know in order to live a full and rich life. Would you tell me those secrets?" The Master bowed in return and said, "Yes, I will tell you. The first secret is pay attention. The second secret is pay attention, and the third secret is pay attention".' (Ray & Myers, 1986, p. 66).

The two quotations above introduce us to the world of reflection—the world where close attention and focus on our work begins the journey of making sense of the experience itself, learning from it and doing it differently. Horton (1990) called this process: *'helping people learn what they do'*.

The medium of learning in supervision is primarily reflective. While tradition and theories gather and garner the reflective experiences of others, reflection is a way to learn personally from the events within our own lives. Supervision is a form of conversation that facilitates learning. Critical reflection allows participants to learn together in dialogue. Isaacs (1999) defines dialogue as a way of *'thinking together in relationship'* and Belenky, Clinchy, Goldberger, & Tarule (1986) draw out what this means:

'In didactic talk, each participant may report experience, but there is no attempt amongst participants to join together to arrive at some new understanding. 'Really talking' requires some careful listening; it implies a mutually shared agreement that together you are creating the optimum setting so that half-baked ideas can grow. 'Real talk' reaches deep into the experience of each participant; it also draws on the analytical abilities of each' (p. 144).

If supervision can be seen as a mini 'community of practice' where dialogue is the form of conversation used and critical reflection allows participants to be open to multiple possibilities, then learning takes place through reflective dialogue which leads to generative action through transformational learning.

There is a distinction between *'reflection'*, which is a focus on the 'what' of experience, e.g., my work, life, relationships, and *'reflectivity'*, which is the process of reflecting on the 'I' who is reflecting. Both are involved in reflective learning.

Introduction

It is only humans in the animal kingdom that have the ability to reflect. Our language is replete with words and phrases showing our propensity to reflect: *"I thought about what you said"*, *"I'll mull it over and we'll talk tomorrow"*, *"What do you think about what he did?"*, *"Why did you do that?"*, *"I caught myself saying"*, *"Let me think some more about it"*. We not only act, but also then think about what we have done. We can even think about our thinking on what we have done. We not only reflect on what we have done, but we reflect on the person who is doing the reflection (if that doesn't sound too convoluted!).

Reflection is a sophisticated skill. Like learning itself, the ability to reflect has much to do with our past and our experience of prior reflection, as well as our personality, environment and the people who surround us in our lives.

What is reflection?

In general, reflection is the *'ability to step back and pose hard questions about: why are things done this way? How could I do it differently?'* Voller (2010) defines and describes reflection as, *'Purposeful focusing on thoughts, feelings, sensations and behaviour in order to make meaning from those fragments of experience. The outcome of this reflection is to create new understanding which in turn may lead to: increasing choices, making changes or reducing confusion'* (p. 21).

The word 'reflection' comes from Latin roots meaning *'to bend back, to stand apart from, to stand outside of'*. In reflection, we take a step back and look at what we or others have done. Reflection means 'stepping back' so that I gain a new perspective on what I have done.

Here are a few more definitions of reflection:

1. *'Reflection is an active, persistent and careful consideration of any belief or supposed form of knowledge in the light of the grounds that support it and the future conclusions to which it leads'* (Dewey, 1933).

2. *'Reflection can be defined as thinking and feeling activities in which individuals engage to explore their experiences in order to lead to new understandings and appreciations'* (Boud, Keogh & Walker, 1985, p. 19).

3. *'Reflection is a process by which I interrogate my own thoughts, feelings and actions'*.

4. *'Reflection is the ability to create meaning and conceptualisation from experience and the potentiality to look at things other than as they are'* (Brockbank & McGill, 1998).

5. *'Reflexivity is the intention to examine one's actions, active and critical inquiry, openness to alternatives and willing to be vulnerable to try out new ideas'* (Neufeldt, 1999).

From these definitions we can see that reflection and reflexivity have a number of common features.

Moon (1999) word associates around the term reflection and comes up with a veritable dictionary of possible substitute words: *'reasoning, thinking, reviewing, problem solving, inquiry, reflective judgement, critical reflection…'* (p. v11). Other animals, while clearly able to learn from experience, do not seem to have that critical facility that allows them to delve deeper into their experience in order to manufacture meaning. Gilbert (2006) puts this humorously when he writes, *'Until a chimp weeps at the thought of growing old alone, or smiles as it contemplates its summer holidays, or turns down a toffee apple because it looks too fat in shorts, I will stand by my version of the sentence which is, the human being is the only animal that thinks about the future'* (p. 4). Reflection is the ability to think about the past, in the present, for the future. As Gilbert also points out, our way to access the future is through imagination.

In the light of the above, reflection has a number of characteristics:

1. Reflection is an 'internal' activity. I harness my thoughts and feelings to consider, thinking about what has happened. I go inside to access my capacity to review what I have done or what has happened. Reflection starts with being able to stop doing and begin thinking about what has transpired.

2. The purpose of the activity is to hold experience 'up to the light', to allow it to speak to me so that I can learn from it.

3. Reflection is a process of examination, inquiry, self-interrogation where I ask questions of the activity itself. Why did this happen? Why did I do that? Why did that person respond in that way? Why do I keep getting into these situations? Reflection can also ask questions of the person reflecting. Who am I who is reflecting? Why do I reflect this way?

4. Reflection is a way of making sense of and giving meaning to events and experiences. Reflection is a way of giving attention and focus to what we already know in order to achieve further insights that lead to further

knowledge. It is a meaning-making facility that helps me understand from a number of perspectives. Widening reflectivity means widening the meaning and making frameworks from which I work.

5. Reflection is not just a rational event—it is an emotional experience as well (Moore, 2008; Moon, 2004).

6. With reflection, I can then look at alternatives, other ways of thinking or doing: *'Reflection requires linking existing knowledge to an analysis of the relationship between current experience and future action'* (McAlpine & Weston, 2002, p. 69).

7. Reflection focuses on processes for which there is no obvious or clear cut solution, no certain knowledge (Moon, 1999, p. 4). Certainty needs no reflection. King and Kitchener (1994) make the distinction between *'well-structured problems'*, which have an answer and often a single answer, and *'ill-structured problems'*, which can have a number of possible answers and often no absolute right answer. Reflection is the process of how people reason about ill-structured problems.

Schon (1983; 1987) talks about two types of reflection: *'reflection-in-action'* and *'reflection-on-action'*. The first type (present tense reflection or the ability to pause in the middle of action) observes and reflects on what we are doing as we are doing it—what Bolton (2001) calls *'the hawk in your mind constantly circling over your head watching and advising on your actions—while you are practicing'* (p. 15). Casement (1985) coined the term *'internal supervisor'* to capture this type of reflection within the area of psychotherapy. He suggested creating *'an island of intellectual contemplation'* (see Henderson, 2009 for a review of the internal supervisor). As we engage with our work, we become our own supervisor, monitoring, thinking, evaluating, and assessing what is going on. It is a way to make sense of what is happening as it is happening. The second kind of reflection, *'recollective reflection'*, is the more luxurious reflection-on-action where we stop activities and intentionally put ourselves into a stance of curiosity and inquiry. We think backwards using a past experience as the focus of our thinking. We are provided with time, space, safety and attention to focus on and think about our experiences. A third type of reflection is *'reflection for action'* (anticipatory reflection) where we prepare for the future using imagination to think through and evaluate possible scenarios.

Exercise

Using some of the definitions above could you take 10 minutes to reflect on something that has happened to you recently? It could be a personal or professional experience. Take notes of what is happening to you during this process.

Learning reflection

How can we move from a non-reflective stance to a reflexive position? Can we learn how to reflect? An external event is not always needed to engender reflection, but for many people (especially those not used to or skilled in reflection) an external happening often propels them into reflection. Facing a problem makes individuals or groups 'ripe for reflection'. And the type of problem faced is 'ill-structured', which means it does not have a single and solitary solution. Uncertainty, confusion and surprise are often emotional pathways to help us reconsider and think through what we have never thought through before. Wake-up calls, high-wire moments, shocks and traumas—all are potential triggers for processes of reflection. They impel us to wonder why, to question, to review our old way of thinking which is inadequate to encompass this new event.

The 'internal' requirements that facilitate our reflections are:

1. Openness and open-mindedness. Rokeach (1979) defines open-mindedness as *'the extent to which a person can receive, evaluate, and act on relevant information received from outside on its own intrinsic merits unencumbered by irrelevant factors in the situation arising from within the person or from outside'* (p. 57). Being honest with oneself, being open to *'whatever truth comes through the door'*, being courageous enough to stay with the facts all greatly assist reflection.

2. Being mindful. *'Mindfulness is a particular, purposeful way of being attentive to internal stages of feelings and thoughts and external states of the environment and behaviours, from one moment to the next, and holding this awareness with an attitude of acceptance'* (May & O'Donovan, 2007, p. 48).

3. Invention and imagination, i.e., the ability to go beyond our own psychological boundaries and parameters and permit ourselves to think other possibilities.

4. The ability to stop, be still, recall, get distance from.

5. Suspending evaluation, become non-evaluative until you have had time to observe and take in all the information.

6. Listening to self and others allows you to make sense of what is happening.

7. A respect for intuition and feelings as guides toward understanding.

8. Thinking as a 'beginner'.

9. Looking for other meanings, e.g., how might others make sense of this?

10. Widening one's perspective.

11. Being vulnerable.

12. Befriending the unfamiliar and the uncomfortable.

13. Being emotionally aware of what is happening to us and to others.

14. The ability to think about and consider events and life in wider perspectives: the helicopter ability. The higher you go up the more you see in context.

Context becomes an important fact in reflection. It allows me to make meaning as part of a particular context. Langer (1989) makes the point that when we ignore context we end up giving one meaning when there may be many. She asks individuals to tell her what she is holding in her hand. *"What is this?"*, she asks, holding up a pencil. When people confine themselves to defining the object as a pencil she then asks, *"What could it be?"*. Of course, there are many things this item we call a pencil could be. By committing ourselves too quickly to its own purpose (a pencil) we can miss the other meanings and uses it might have. She makes the point that while defining a pencil may be innocuous and innocent, what happens when we define a family, or a person? Committing ourselves to one meaning of family can close us off to seeing other meanings of the word and give rise to prejudice or stereotyping.

Blocks to reflection

Blocks to reflection can also be internal or external. Being stressed, tired, exhausted, makes reflection very difficult—the mind is too weary or the opposite, too preoccupied. In our 'world of high speed', it is often impossible to get quality reflection time. Some people cannot be 'still', either physically or psychologically, again making reflection difficult. Perhaps today we have to move more towards 'reflection-in-action', where the very speed of life means we need to learn to contemplate quickly as we engage in activity. Our society's glorification of 'action' and 'outcomes' can often result in poor support for reflective activity because 'the point of it' is not billable or rewarded; organisations do not build it into work time. Personality types may also affect the need and the ability to reflect, and whether one is introverted or extroverted may indicate ease or not with reflection-in-action and reflection-on-action.

'*Premature cognitive commitment*' is a term coined by Langer (1989) where, too quickly and without reflection, we commit ourselves to an embedded belief which then impacts our behaviour. With commitment to a belief, we easily give up reflection. She gives the example of how the Ugly Duckling first committed itself to the cognitive belief that it was a duck, and second, that it was ugly. With experience and reflection on its experience came a realisation about who it truly was and subsequently, its self esteem. Premature cognitive commitments mean we often move too quickly to conclusions that are unwarranted when more reflection and attention to the facts might result in different conclusions. She includes classification systems in this mindless approach to reality: '*Mindlessness sets in when we rely too rigidly on categories and distinctions created in the past. Once distinctions are made they take on a life of their own*' (p. 11). Hence the fact that many lead unreflective lives, even when their lives are based on deep commitments. Siegel (2007) captures this well, '*As we grow into adulthood, it is very likely that these accumulated layers of perceptual models and conceptual categories constrict subjective time and deaden our feelings of being alive. Without the intentional effort to awaken, life speeds by. We habituate to experience, perceiving through the filter of the past and not orientating ourselves to the novel distinctions of the present*' (p. 105). Included in the above is a warning about being too certain or committed to a theory or an orientation. Such a stance can lead too easily to premature conclusions or predetermined positions.

The brain is excellent at creating patterns and classification systems. It sets down neural pathways that become habitual ways of perceiving and when new information enters the system it is compared and contrasted with the old classification systems. The first task of the brain is to make the new information fit the old system. The brain is, in fact, quite lazy and sees little reason in wasting valuable energy in considering or finding arguments to reject perfectly well-formed beliefs (classifications systems). Fine (2007) calls this the 'Pigheaded Brain' and shows with colour and humour how we hold onto our beliefs and classification systems even when overwhelming evidence shows the contrary. '*Evidence that fits with our beliefs*', she writes, '*is quickly waved through the mental border control. Counter-evidence on the other hand, must submit to close interrogation and even then will probably not be allowed in*' (p. 106).

Expectations are a further way of blocking our reflection. Unconscious or unspoken expectations impair out ability to reflect. The psychological contract (our internal interpretation of the contracts we have in our lives) often impairs this ability to reflect, e.g., the expectation of a teenager that they will not be liked by their peer group often muddies their ability to think about what the group does and its usefulness (taking drugs, using alcohol, etc.). Loyalty (that becomes collusion) impacts the ability to reflect.

Fear and living in survival mode greatly reduces reflection and the ability to make meaning. In general, when fear and anxiety are high, individuals interpret the events in their lives in narrow ways, e.g., going into victim mode and blaming others. Another emotion that has a negative effect on our ability to reflect and how we reflect is 'shame'. Individuals and groups who come from shame-based backgrounds (either shame-based family systems of shame-based education systems) find it extremely difficult to allow themselves to be vulnerable without being shamed yet again.

Shame is a process that can interfere with learning. When we experience shame, we want to hide away and protect ourselves rather than enter into dialogue. If we enter a shame-based place, we may hesitate to admit to ourselves or others that we need help or support in learning. Many people have had shaming experiences in the course of their schooling where they have been shamed and humiliated for 'not knowing'. As a consequence, they may have learnt to hide their needs and shut down on their natural right to be informed and ask for information. Trust may have been severely undermined in relation to the learning environment. As supervisees we may bring a history of this kind to the supervisory relationship. An educational history of this nature has often left people believing there is only one 'right' way of doing things and that lies in the hands of the 'authority', and different options, points of view and ways of doing things are not acceptable. It is important to raise fears and doubts of this kind in order to have a good supervisory relationship (see Gilbert & Evans, 2000, for a discussion of shame in supervision). We recommend a supervisory contract in which mutual respect for each other's points of view is a ground rule as is a clear understanding that this is a co-operative relationship!

Kaufman (1992), in his exploration of shame, writes of the mutuality that is central to our feeling secure in a real relationship with another. *'The bond which ties two individuals together forms an interpersonal bridge between them'* (Kaufmann 1992, p. 13). In this process of mutuality we can permit ourselves to receive respect and valuing from the other. Such an atmosphere of trust provides a facilitative environment for learning to take place. This interpersonal bridge is built on certain expectations of a relationship that will be influenced by our past experience of rewarding relationships in general and will, of course, be impacted significantly by the respectful approach of people to us in the present.

If someone ridicules us and our struggles, the interpersonal bridge will be broken by this rupture in the relationship. If this has happened to us repeatedly in past learning situations, we may experience a reluctance to open up to new learning in the present especially where our need is great and we feel a reluctance to admit to vulnerability and the need for help. However, should we experience shame in a supervisory relationship, however inadvertent this may be on the part of the supervisor, it will be important to open up the discussion and mend the rupture in the relationship for further learning to occur. Someone who does not know our history may sometimes put ideas into a form of words that we find difficult because of past experience. Such misunderstandings are good to discuss and clarify otherwise this will stand in the way of further learning until the trust has been re-established in the relationship. Kaufman (1992) speaks of this process as healing the interpersonal bridge between people; this can serve as a powerful reparative process in the present especially where shame-based learning has occurred in the past. We can then move forward with the learning process.

Reflection, in being transparent about what can be known, means permitting the self to be open to disconfirm what is already known and what is not known. These mental stances can be difficult to take on for people from shame-based backgrounds. In admitting or owning their ignorance, doubts, uncertainties they leave themselves open to not living up to their own or others' expectations. This then plunges them, as it did in the past, into a shame-based place which closes them down and makes them want to withdraw. For them, learning to reflect in an open way often involves having a relationship they can trust not to shame them and being able to take the risks of being vulnerable. It is quite a relational journey when shame raises its ugly head.

Given that part of reflection is the ability to be creative and imaginative, lack of creativity and 'outside the box' thinking is a further block to reflection. Gilbert (2006) reminds us that we access the future through imagination. Reflection is also a way to access the future. When our ability to access imagination (for whatever reason) is limited, then we tend to act in predictable and mindless routines.

In 'The Curse of the Self', Leary (2004) considers the drawbacks of reflection. While a blessing and a highly human activity, there are times when reflection becomes our enemy, not our friend. It is more helpful to be mindless and unreflective when I am trying to get to sleep. Too much reflection, often called rumination, keeps many people awake at night or rouses them early in the morning when their reflective minds refuse to allow them to go back to sleep. Worry, which is a form of reflecting on the future, is equally troublesome at the times when we get so caught up in our reflective concerns for the future that we miss what is happening in the present. It is good that we don't have to reflect on how we drive our cars, dress ourselves in the morning, manage our PCs or do the shopping. We do these tasks automatically. For actions and behaviours that do not demand creativity or imagination going onto automatic pilot suits very well.

Over-reflection has drawbacks in that it:

1. Interferes with memory.
2. Puts us out of touch with what we already know.
3. Disconnects us from cognitive processes (if you think too much about the presentation you are about to give it may well result in choking).
4. Can result in poorer performance.
5. Can result in mental illnesses (compulsions, depressions, etc.).
6. Can result in unhelpful behaviour (there is some evidence from surveys of teenage girls that they often smoke as a way of staying thin—the desire to be seen as beautiful makes them take a risk with their health).

The inner world of animals does not include the self-related thoughts of humans. But we humans talk to ourselves. People live in their inner worlds when there is no need to, and even when it pulls them away from attending to life in the external world.

What helps reflection?

A number of factors impact on the ability to reflect. Prior experiences are one. Families and schools that encourage children to reflect and think through issues can dramatically affect their ability to reflect later in life. Where children grow up in environments that teach them certainties around ill-structured problems, they learn easily not to think but to instead accept the words of authorities. Students bring their pasts with them to their new experiences and how well they reflect and integrate these new experiences into their lives depends to a large degree on those experiences.

King and Kitchener (1994) make a number of suggestions of how to help people learn how to reflect:

1. Show respect for individuals as people regardless of their level of development.

2. Understand that individuals differ regarding their assumptions about knowledge and personalise your interventions: *'When their responses are dogmatic, I foster all their doubts; when they seem mired in skepticism or paralysed by complexity, I push them to make judgements; when their tactics are not fully reflective, I encourage their best efforts to use critical, evaluative thinking'* (Kroll, 1992, as cited in King & Kitchener, 1994, p. 232).

3. Introduce 'ill-structured problems' early and encourage individuals to wrestle with them.

4. Create opportunities for students to examine different points of view on a topic.

5. Help students suspend judgement temporarily.

6. Help individuals make judgements and explain what they believe.

7. Provide lots of support and lots of challenge.

8. Deal with the emotional aspects of learning and realise that much reflection is the ability to understand, name and manage emotional reactions. Big emotions (e.g., shame) can be very detrimental to facilitating reflection.

Langer (1989) suggests a number of ways to help develop mindfulness and reflection:

1. Creating new categories helps us see old ideas in new ways.

2. Welcoming new information.

3. Realising and appreciating more than one view.

4. Controlling contexts—allowing the context to teach us.

5. Process before outcomes (from journey to 'destinational' learning).

There is no doubt that questions are a key way in which to facilitate reflection. The right question jolts, goes to the heart of the matter, surprises, makes the listener realise that their solutions to date no longer work with this issue. Reflective questions lead to insight. Kagan's IPR (1980) is an excellent way to assist reflection. See also Appendices 18 and 20 at the back of this manual for lists of incisive and reflective questions.

One way to facilitate reflection is to help learners find their own voice (Belenky et al., 1986). Voicing reflections helps encourage reflection—there is some truth in the statement that I do not know what I know until I have said it, or written it down. Giving feedback is another way to help individuals to begin to reflect.

In summary, individuals learn to reflect at ever-deepening levels when they:

1. Learn how to be empathic and see events from other perspectives.
2. Are confused in their thinking.
3. Begin to look at the consequences of their behaviour.
4. Monitor and articulate their feelings.
5. Are challenged to look at what they are doing and why they are doing it.
6. Ask incisive questions.
7. Create connections to others.
8. Specifically go out to meet others who are different and think differently.
9. Are shocked.
10. Move towards authenticity and congruence.
11. Begin to self-disclose.
12. Build up their thinking skills.
13. Stop.
14. Are prepared to experiment.
15. Use counselling, training or courses to review how they reflect.
16. Are allowed to change roles.
17. Befriend the uncomfortable and unfamiliar.
18. Put themselves in challenging (stretching) situations.
19. Live with groups that think differently.

Reflection is too important to be left to chance. Too much depends on it to hope that it might be picked up during the journey of life. Rather, it seems wiser to teach or facilitate how to reflect, so that individuals and groups can be assured of having such a precious commodity. While facilitating reflection here has been defined as an individual task, there is no doubt that helping people reflect in groups is a very valuable way to help individuals.

The process of reflection

A number of areas come together to make the process or stages that reflection goes through possible. The following is not meant to be a rigid step-by-step process of reflection but can be seen as an overview of the steps reflection goes through. Figure 15 summarises the stages and steps of the model:

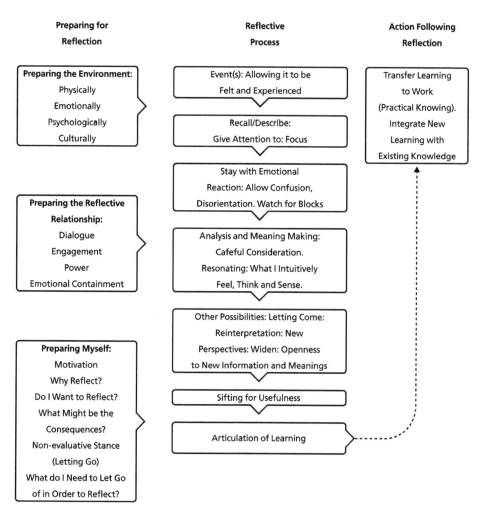

Figure 15: The Process of Reflection

We can use Figure 15 not only as a model for focusing on reflective practice, but also as a figure to help us take a step back and look at the process by which reflection takes place—reflection-on-reflection (what we earlier called reflexivity, looking at the person doing the reflection).

We can now look at the stages outlined in Figure 15.

Preparing for reflection

Three factors need to be in place before reflection can take place: a) preparing the environment for reflection—physical, emotional, psychological and cultural preparation; b) preparing of the reflective relationship and the components involved in that relationship, and; c) preparing myself by reviewing and consolidating my motivation and taking a non-evaluative stance that permits wide reflection.

Clearing a space to help the reflective process is important. Being in the right frame of mind helps enormously. It is here that some of the research on mindfulness can help. Put simply, mindfulness is learning to be fully alert and available in the present moment (Carroll, 2004). Mindfulness is also a purposeful way of being attentive to internal states of feelings and thoughts, as well as external states of the environment (May & O'Donovan, 2007). It helps us to remain attentive without judgement. Siegel (2007) recommends silence as one method of setting up mindfulness and reflection, *'silence creates a rare opportunity to pause and drop into stillness, to become intimate with your own mind. When we start the journey to attune to our own minds by pausing into stillness we enter a new realm of experience that can produce surprise in each moment'* (p. 72).

Siegel also suggests that meditation is a good method to create stillness and focus the mind. He quotes research by Lazar which concludes that meditation might alter the very structures of our brains that are responsible for empathy and for self-observation (p. 104). Relaxed, alert and focused we are ready to reflect. Creating the best physical environment, preparing ourselves emotionally to be reflective, awareness of our psychological helps and blocks with regard to setting up an ideal reflective environment, and being alert to cultural issues, all help us get ready for the process called reflection.

The relationship/s which surround us (the supervisory, counselling or coaching relationship) are a second factor in preparing the reflective ground. How power is used in the relationship, the kind of engagement involved and the type of conversation used all contribute to the atmosphere of reflection (or not, as the case may be). How contained we feel emotionally is a further factor in our readiness to allow ourselves the vulnerability of reflection.

The third preparatory factor is the ability to monitor our motivation and get ourselves into a non-judgemental stance. Scharmer (2007) describes the latter well, *'But it is only in the suspension of judgement that we can open ourselves up to wonder. Wonder is about noticing that there is a world beyond our patterns of downloading... without the capacity for wonder, we will most likely remain stuck in the prison of our mental constructs'* (p. 134). The reason why we reflect is equally important and worth articulating for ourselves.

Doing reflection

Ready to reflect, we now turn our focus and attention to experience, in the case of supervision, our work, and begin to immerse ourselves in the remembered events. We allow our work into our minds, we become sensitive to what happened, we observe, notice, take stock of, perceive and look at in detail. Leonardo da Vinci used to send his students to study a fish and draw it. On their return, he would tell them to go back and look again. He repeated this process with them many times based on the principle that there are always new perceptions we have missed or overlooked.

This stage in the reflective process could be called 'Attention'. Siegel (2007) divides Attention into three parts: *'alerting'* (involving attention, vigilance and alertness); *'orienting'* (selecting certain information from a variety of options to scan or select); and *'executive attention'* (which is about our intention to sift and control the process) (p. 113). We recollect, describe and tell the story: What happened? Describe the event. Don't evaluate it. Remember it. Perceive it again, and again. Look at it anew. What are you missing, what are you not seeing? Huston (2007) connects attention and judgement, *'The act of pure observation occurs without judgement...we must dispense with judgement based on past experience and simply observe what is, what is actually said or done, what is seen, heard, smelled, tasted or touched...it is the act of the discipline attention that allows us to notice things we sometimes overlook'* (p. 97).

We stay with our feelings and emotions and allow ourselves to think with feeling. We permit the confusions, the disorientation, the fears, the joys, the anxieties and whatever other emotions impact us. Moore (2008) sees supervision as the place where supervisees are offered space to explore the empathic impact that work with clients has had on them. *'The supervisee'*, he writes, *'requires a high degree of self awareness to differentiate between those feelings arising from her own experiences and those given to her in empathy...exploring the emotional impact in depth and applying her theoretical understanding helps the supervisee to make sense of her own emotions and gain insight into the client's dilemmas'* (p. 51).

Our next move involves making sense of what we have focused on. We now give meaning to what happened. We tell a story that embodies our way of making meaning (the process) and the meaning itself (the content). Having focused, sifted, observed, looked again, we conclude and assess and evaluate what we experienced. This involves looking at our feelings, being in touch with our thoughts and observing our behaviours. We monitor these feelings: What were you thinking and feeling? Any reasons why you were thinking and feeling this way? Any connections to the past? Voller (2010) uses the word 'resonance' to capture this moment—where feelings, thoughts, intuitions, discernments, body awareness and musing all come together.

We now widen our reflective stance to consider other meanings. We go wider and more in-depth. If we looked previously at what story we tell, we now review other stories we could tell. We can even look at the way we construct our stories. We look at how we make meaning to see if the very way we have drawn our conclusions means we have missed other ways of making meaning (e.g., we have downloaded experience rather than allowing it to speak to us, we come with a prejudiced mind, we have categories that entrap us). This sometimes demands suspending our judgement once more to allow other voices to be heard. We become empathic to other theories, other people, and other approaches. We let go in order to let come (Scharmer, 2007). We allow our intuitions, imaginations, and creative thoughts and feelings to enter the frame. With analysis we ask further questions: *How do you make sense of what happened? Any other ways of making sense of it?* Be creative—think of another possible interpretation of the experience.

We sift and assess our new insights with our original ideas and thoughts. We evaluate for usefulness. We reach conclusions. We connect our original experiences with our new ways of making meaning and sense of them. We ask evaluative questions: *In your view what was good and bad about the experience? What was helpful and unhelpful?*

We begin to articulate our learning. We have looked at, given meaning to, critically evaluated how we have given meaning to, and looked at other meanings and sense-making procedures, and now we draw our conclusions. Possibilities: *What else could you have done?* Voller (2010) puts this well in asking questions: *What new knowledge or learning has come through to me? What am I taking away from reflection in term of insights, feelings, thoughts? How can I integrate what I have learned into my existing frameworks and knowledge? How can I make my learning part of myself? Overall, what have I learned from that experience, about myself? About others? About work and practice?*

The third stage is the transfer of reflective knowing into action. The bridge between reflection and action transfers new learning (propositional or declarative knowing) into behaviour (transformational learning). The action plan can be helped by answering questions such as: *What will you do differently when you return to that situation? If you were to encounter that again, what would you do?*

Levels of reflection (on learning reflection)

Reflection is a key component in learning (Moon, 1999; 2004). Being able to reflect on our lives and our work is crucial if we are not to fall into mindlessness, the routine process of doing the same things over and over again. Other animals, besides humans, live mindless lives driven mostly by instincts with little ability to reflect on why they do what they do. My attempts to teach our cat to reflect end in frustration for me and cat-boredom for him. He has no ability to make sense of his life or ascribe meaning to why he does certain behaviours, e.g., kill little birds when he is well-fed, capture and play with mice when he has every reason for being more loving, or beat up the cat next door when a little good neighbourliness would go a long way to establishing peace. He cannot change his behaviour through a process of reflection, e.g., decide to diet a little when he puts on a few pounds, change his sleeping patterns, etc. Cami (his name) has no ability to hold his life up to the light and ponder its meaning. He cannot access his 'inner kitten' and work on his self-awareness. The reason, of course, why he cannot reflect is due to the fact that he has a very small frontal cortex in his brain. Unlike us humans who have much larger frontal cortices, executive or human brains as they are sometimes called, Cami is condemned to living an unreflected life. It was Socrates who remarked that such a life is not worth living though he was probably referring to humans, not cats.

Reflection is our human way of making meaning in life (Mezirow, Taylor, & Associates, 2009). Reflection is the bridge between information and wisdom: more, it's the process that turns information and knowledge into wisdom. Through reflection, reflexiveness, and critical thinking, the events of our lives make sense for us and give us choices about how to infuse these events with meanings we choose, rather than meanings that are chosen for us. We are meaning-making animals and it remains very important for us to make sense of our lives by pondering on the events that go to make them up. Telling stories is one way—we narrate our lives as a method of making sense of them for ourselves and to communicate the meaning we have made to others.

However, our ways of making meaning can be very narrow and rigid. Some individuals have only one way to make meaning, e.g., interpreting everything that happens to them through a victim stance. Others have diverse and multiple ways of making sense of events in their lives, e.g., *"Yes, I was partially responsible for the heart attack because of my life style, it has been a wake-up call for me and it's a message about changing some behaviours in my life"*. Some of our helping strategies involve us in supporting others to give different or new meaning to the events in their lives. Counselling is a way of changing the meaning of events—clearly not the historical events themselves. What previously has been given the meaning of being a tragedy, e.g., a divorce or an illness, can be re-interpreted and given new meaning as a 'new start' or a new way of appreciating life. Coaching too is often a way of helping coachees make sense of their lives and their work and, at times, to adopt new perspectives on what they are and what they do.

Supervision is particularly strong on helping supervisees look again at their work and see it from other perspectives. It is a process about a way of looking at what we do and how: with super–vision, new eyes, new perceptions, new visions we can see things differently. Supervision is about a new way of looking, a super way of visioning. With new visions come new perspectives and new meanings. I notice new things. Supervision is always about the quality of awareness. With reflection comes meaning at different levels. As I step outside my comfort zone and take an open stance, without judgement or shame, without blame or assumption, and am open and indifferent to the outcome, what would I allow myself to think and reflect upon? Can I look beyond, beside, beneath, above, below, against, for? What would happen if I looked at myself, my client, our relationship, the organisation in another way?

Supervision is about paying attention to our practice. It is the dancing partner of our work (Murphy, 2009). We stop doing, we pull back from our work, and we start thinking/reflecting. We move from subject, where we are identified with or attached to our work, to object where we can take a perspective outside ourselves. We move from reflection-in-action to reflection-on-action to reflection-for-action. Supervision is a strategic withdrawal to meditate, contemplate, and think about our work. In the attention to and the reflection on, we learn how to do our work differently and better. This is the purpose of supervision: it is a 'respectful interruption' of our work to set up reflective dialogues through which we learn from the very work we do. The medium we do this through is reflection—reflection becomes the method through which we learn. Reflection is the discipline of wondering about…what if?

Reflection fits within the larger picture of experiential learning (Kolb, 1984). Marsick and Maltbia (2009) have used the ORID model—*Objective, Reflective, Interpretative* and *Decisive* data—to illustrate how experimental learning works. We have added a further section to this model, an Integrative arm. Table 2 outlines the process under a number of headings:

ELC	Process	Focus	Method
Action	Objective	What Happened? Is Happening?	Observe Facts, Events. Notice, Give Attention.
Reflection	Reflective	What am I Feeling? What is My Reaction?	Monitor and Articulate Reactions
Reflection	Interpretative	What Does it Mean?	Utilise Critical Thinking
Learning	Integrative	What Have I Learned?	Assimilate into New Learning
Application	Decisive	What do I do?	Implement Decisions

Table 2: The Experimental Learning Cycle

Our focus here is the Reflective/Interpretative sections of this model and the reflective section of the Experiential Learning Cycle. If reflection is so important for us, then why isn't it taught more? As far as we know there are few lessons or training programmes in reflection, how to reflect, deepening reflection and using reflection to make sense of life.

Recently, we have been working on how to understand reflection (Carroll, 2009) and, in particular, how to help coachees and supervisees use reflection to its maximum. As a result we have devised six modes or levels of reflection that allow us to look at the same event from six perspectives and make meaning in six different ways using reflection as the medium of learning. There is no magic in having six levels, there may well be more. By adopting six possible viewpoints each taking six different viewpoints we can get a 360 degree perspective and can use these insights to create the best possible interventions. Table 3 below provides a brief summary of the six levels and later we will use an example to illustrate how the six levels can be used. Have a look also at Appendix 19 which summarises the descriptions of the six levels below.

Level	Ability for Reflection	Stance/Attitude	Connection Quality
1	Zero	Me	Disconnected
2	Empathic	Observer	Empathic Connection
3	Relational	You and Me = Us	Personal Connection
4	Systemic	You and Me + Others	Contextual Connection
5	Self-reflection	Me (Internalised)	Incorporating Connection
6	Transcendental	Other (Universal)	Universal Connection

Table 3: Levels of Reflection, Stances and Connectivity

Each level is presented below using the same six general categories:

1. Description of the level.
2. The TA (Transactional Analysis) Position it tends to adopt.
3. Typical statements made from this position.
4. What the end result might be.
5. The strategy that seems to characterise this reflective stance.
6. What blocks us from moving to the next level of reflection?

Have a look at Appendix 19 where we have put this in a more organised way.

Level 1: Zero reflection (me-stance, disconnection)

Level one is a non-reflective stance: *"I am right, you are way off the mark"*. This level of reflection finds it difficult to go internal or look at wider pictures or bigger systems. It has an either-or stance to making sense of events and is based on a theory of causality that is very simple, such as 'this caused that to happen'. There is no awareness of circular causality here, of where cause and effect intertwine. The answer we seek is usually quite straight forward: *"If you would change, my life would be easier"*.

1. **Positions:** I'm ok (could be I'm not ok), you're not ok. A position of blame is often adopted. This can easily be a victim stance—*"See how badly the world treats me!"* We call this the 'me-stance (external)' because it focuses on the actor/person but from an external perspective—there is little consideration for how I might be part of the problem or contribute to it. By and large at this stage: *"You are the problem, I am the solution"*.

2. **Statements we make:** *"This client is resistant... This coachee is not committed to the process... This manager wants to get her own way... This leader cannot delegate because of his issues with power... Because it is obvious, that's the way it is"*.

3. **Result:** Stuckness, strong feeling and often negative resentment. Individuals here often stay solely at the content (not process) level, or have a simplistic answer to life.

4. **Strategy** is one of telling or asserting as if it were totally true: *"This is what you will do or should do"*. The conversation is one of monologue. There can be detachment, withdrawal or defensiveness here too.

5. **Blocks to further reflection:** Being certain, being right, very strong feelings, fear of giving up control and power. Fear and shame are further blocks at this level.

Level 2: Empathic reflection (observer stance, connections)

Level 2 reflection sees the reflector beginning to become more of an observer with acknowledgement of feelings. There is a movement from event to personality. There is an awareness of some empathy for the perspective of the other or for another perspective. A more compassionate interpretation allows for insights into what is happening to the other.

1. **Positions:** I'm ok (could still be I'm not ok) and realising you might be ok (but not yet). You are still the problem and I am still, by and large the solution. A position of blame plus understanding (some empathy) is most common.
2. **Statements we make:** *"I can understand why the person does this, although that does not excuse it…I must be more understanding, but hold the line …I can be somewhat accommodating now that I understand what is happening".*
3. **Result:** More understanding and loosening of response. The certainty that comes with Level 1 has begun to unfreeze.
4. **Strategy:** I still tell/force what to do. Conversation can be discussion or debate or still be monologue.
5. **Blocks to deeper reflection:** Not believing I contribute to this, not wanting to give control and power, simplistic causality thinking. Still elements of being certain or right or of having found the answer.

Level 3: Relational reflection (you-and-me = us stance, personal connection)

Level 3 often follows a dialogue (internal or external) where we begin to share the issues and start to see that many of the issues or problems are relational (now I see that it is about you and me, and how we are getting on or not together). We begin to see that the issue, the problem, what we are facing, is in fact relational rather than simply part of one person. While we both bring our personal histories into this shared space there is awareness that we create a relational dilemma for which we both have some responsibility. We can work out a way of working together.

1. **Position:** We are ok if we can talk about it. Position is one of collective responsibility. An 'us' stance. We have a problem, we have the solution.
2. **Statements we make:** *"Let's talk about this…How do you think we both contribute to the issue/s?…What can we do together to make this situation more manageable for both of us?…How can I begin to see this from multiple*

perspectives?... Where are the connections?... How do we 'make' this problem together?"

3. **Result:** Movement from projecting, blaming and seeing the problem located in another to seeing that we co-create the issue.

4. **Strategy:** We talk honestly and openly about ourselves, our needs and our relationship. Self-awareness allows other information into the system, e.g., my need to control. Reflective dialogue (where together we begin to think about and talk about the issues) is used.

5. **Blocks to further reflection:** The problem is solved; no awareness of psychological patterns in my life. Denial because of the work I would have to do if I believed there is another level of refection. The problem is in the system. Or little awareness that the wider systems to which we belong impact on us and co-create the problem with us.

Level 4: Systemic reflection (contextual connection)

This is the systemic reflective stance that looks to the system and the various subsystems involved and allows us to reflect on the situation from these perspectives. It is the helicopter (or satellite) ability to see the various small and large systems that affect our lives and our behaviours. Level 4 reflection looks for the connections between the 'you' and 'me' that create a larger 'us' extending beyond our immediate dyad, team or group to what shared resources and history shape and influence our choices and values. Level 4 can extend our reflective inquiry into ancestry, heritage, community, culture, ecosystem, etc.

1. **Position:** We're ok. Position is one of systemic responsibility. The bigger picture stance. How is it all connected and how can we see and reflect from these multiple perspectives?

2. **Statements we make:** *"How do we all contribute to creating a common culture around values that may or may not be conscious but can have immense power to influence our behaviour?... Can I see patterns and themes that impact me, my relationships and my life?... How does our communal stance create this kind of situation?"*

3. **Result:** Taking a larger view that considers the various systems levels (culture, politics, values, gender, discourse and dominant narratives, etc.).

4. **Strategy:** Reflect on system as affecting behaviour. What do we need to be aware of and change in order for this situation to be different? Creating external generative dialogue that results in action. Moving to upstream

helping rather than downstream resuscitation, i.e., seeing the system as a problem and not just the individual.

5. **Blocks to further reflection:** See the big picture, but forget about individuals.

Level 5: Self-reflection (me-stance, internal, incorporating feedback)

This is the self transcendent position that means I begin to look at me and how I can so easily set up these situations with which I find myself involved (Gosh!, it's actually about me!). It looks at how insight and awareness by me on me can result in ways of working that mean changing my mind set and my meaning making perspectives. I can change, and if I change then others have the opportunity to experience ourselves and the situation differently. Thinking intersubjectively (relationality) but in a way that helps me see my part in this.

1. **Position:** I'm ok, you're ok. Position is one of personal responsibility. The me-stance (internal). I have issues and problems I need to resolve. Unlike Level 1 which is also a 'me' position but external to me, Level 5 goes internal to articulate my own patterns and themes that contribute to the way I engage in life and relationships.

2. **Statements we make:** *"What is my contribution to this?…Can I see patterns in my life whereby I end up here a lot?…How does my way of thinking result in this kind of situation?…What strategies did I develop back-there that still impact my here-and-now behaviour?"*

3. **Result:** I become self aware—aware of myself as person, myself in relationship to others, myself at work. I look for more awareness and insights into myself as agent.

4. **Strategy:** Reflect on self as agent. What do I need to change in order for this situation to be different and for a psychological pattern to be broken? An internal dialogue. I look for the assumptions I bring to life and work, I review my meaning-making processes. I change the thinking behind my thinking.

5. **Blocks to further reflection:** Navel gazing. So caught up in my own development that I forget others. Over-reflection that results in rumination and obsessions. Our inner defences can also become an obstacle to further reflection.

Level 6: Transcendent reflection (transpersonal—connection with the larger)

This is the reflective stance that sees beyond...to what makes meaning and what gives meaning to life. It transcends any particular relationship, person or situation, opening into a larger construct that is inherent in all relationships, people, or situations. For many this can be a religious or spiritual stance that helps reflect from a philosophy or a system of meaning that already exists (e.g., Christianity, Judaism) or one that I create (my philosophy of life). It can be seen as what gives meaning to life, people and behaviour, e.g., that God loves us, that suffering exists, that individuals have value in themselves. It adopts an existential position on life, and is often called the *'Transpersonal'* or *'Transcendent'*. It can be theistically based or not.

1. **Position:** There is a higher or larger perspective that helps me make sense of life and purpose (humanistic, atheistic, denominational religion, Buddhist, etc.). I find meaning by subscribing to this existential position and I attempt to live the current situation through this expanded perspective, recognising my own personal limitations of perception, but with the clear intention to expand my 'little self' and embody more of the qualities of transcendence that guide, teach and inspire me. I am willing to adopt this expanded view/state of being, even though it may require me to enter a space of 'not knowing' and may engender a profound restructuring of my mental constructs.

2. **Statements we make:** *"From within this viewpoint (my philosophy of life) how can I make sense of this event?... What are the real values that I believe in?"* (Sartre, 2003: look at a person's choices and you will see their values).

3. **Result:** Building my behaviour on principles I believe in, that go beyond myself and others as individuals and even systems.

4. **Strategy:** Reflect on life, people and behaviour from a spiritual and transcendent purpose that is bigger than we are. How do I/we reflect from a wider purpose bigger than us all? We find humility, curiosity and reverence helpful here. Finding the over-arching meaning that makes sense of how I/we make meaning.

5. **Blocks to further reflection:** 'So heavenly minded that no earthly good'. Get lost in philosophy or transcendental (rather than an incarnational) theology or spirituality. Get overwhelmed by the vastness of perspective and disconnect from the ordinary delights of daily living. Level 6 can become a flight from reflection and, indeed, a way to avoid reflection.

Example

The following example will illustrate how the six levels might be used in a chronological manner in a coaching situation.

Sarah (who works for Coach Supreme) has been coaching Edward (who works for Maximum Investments, a branch of Allied Continental Banks). The main focus of their executive coaching has been Ed's lack of assertiveness at work and his skills (or lack of them to be more precise) in managing his team. Feedback to Ed has been consistent and ongoing: he needs be more decisive and he needs to deal with the dysfunctional elements in the team. Six months into the coaching (where improvement has been noted by all the players in the system), Ed is made redundant. This has come as a shock to both him and Sarah. He has asked Maximum Investments if Sarah can continue to coach him during this transition time (he has been given a generous allowance for Outplacement Counselling). Sarah knows and has worked with the six level model of reflection and thinks it might help Ed come to accept being made redundant, learn from it and move with more confidence into the next job.

Level 1: Zero-reflection, me-stance: disconnection

Sarah allows Ed to ventilate his feelings of anger, betrayal and abandonment by Maximum Investments. He is very negative, very let down. *"How can they do this to me"*, he exclaims, *"after all I have done for them"*. Ed focuses his feelings on the Company and blames them for not giving the coaching more time to work, for breaking their promises and for not supporting their employees. At this time he is locked into his own feelings and his victim-stance and cannot reflect more widely. There is only one villain in this piece—the Company and the way they deal with employees. Sarah is aware that Ed is locked into Level 1 and strong emotions that are not allowing him to reflect at deeper levels. She knows also that she cannot hurry him along to a new level before he has expressed his feelings and feels he has been heard. She listens and encourages his expressions of feeling.

Level 2: Empathic, observer stance: connections

Very gently and slowly (still allowing for the negative feelings to emerge), Sarah begins to ask Ed to look at why he thinks the Company (Maximum Investments) have made him redundant. Reluctant at first to contemplate such a stance, slowly Ed begins to put himself in the shoes of the organisation and particularly his boss and the HR director and allows himself to access their perspectives. He knows there are redundancies in the company. He knows his recent appraisals have been poor; he knows he has been in his job for only nine months. Despite his resentments, he can understand why they might make him redundant. He still thinks it was untimely and handled badly, but he has allowed himself to view his redundancy from another position and perspective.

Level 3: Relational, you-and-me stance: personal connection

Sarah now asks Ed to see if he can reflect on what has happened (his redundancy) from within a relational perspective. She asks him to look in turn at his relationship with his boss, with the HR director and with the Company in general. Ed notes, in particular, that his relationship with Emily, his boss, was one of dependency. He expected more support and coaching from her. On the other hand, as he reflects back he realises that her expectations of him were that he would be autonomous, independent and only use her when problems arose. He realises they never actually talked about their expectations of each other and never looked at how their relationship was affecting him and his work. Sarah has him talk to Emily (not really but in the coaching room) about these expectations and about their relationship in general. From this, Ed becomes aware that they have both contributed to the relationship and by not talking sooner allowed things to develop to where it became increasingly difficult to discuss with strong and negative feelings on both their parts.

Level 4: Systemic stance: contextual connection

From the platform of relations at work, Sarah helped Ed look at the whole system of Maximum Investments. It is a fast-paced, dynamic organisation that had little time for reflection and is highly action-oriented. It worked on an unspoken rule that if you could not maintain the pace then you fell behind and usually dropped out but no-one was going to carry you. It was an organisation that expected you to survive on your own and not be vulnerable. This culture permeated all its departments. Ed realised that he was out of his depth in this system, not keeping up but afraid to appear to be vulnerable and ask for help. He becomes more aware that the organisational culture emerges in its values and choices and that all the participants are affected by it, for better or worse. He realises that this type of organisational system does not suit him very well and he decided at this stage he will, if need be, give up some salary for more supportive relationships at work.

Level 5: Me-stance, internal: connections, feedback

Ed had widened his ways of reflection and had allowed himself to move from a blame stance to understanding the system within which he had worked. Now, Sarah moves back inwards with him asking, *"What have you learned about yourself from this, Ed.?"* This was a difficult question for Ed but he took it on board and with Sarah's help began to look at how he contributed to what had happened. He realised there were patterns in his life that emerged in his teamwork. He hated conflict of any kind (and he could see where this came from) and so he rarely intervened when conflict situations diverted the focus and the energy of his team. He had lost two good members from that team because he had not intervened to manage the destructive team dynamics. He also saw another psychological pattern in this life—his anxieties about making unilateral decisions and getting it wrong often made him indecisive and made him look tentative and unsure. Sarah remembers his words, *"I need to work on these before I get my next job, otherwise I will take them with me into the next Company".* Much of the rest of the coaching centred on these deep set themes in Ed's life.

Level 6: Transcendental: connections with the larger

In her work with Ed it was obvious to Sarah that his Christian faith meant a lot to him. Several times he had talked about it and its importance in his life and work. As they neared the end of their work together, Sarah asked Ed if there were any other areas he needed to work with before moving on. He said he was still angry and resentful about the way his redundancy had been handled even though now he could see why it was decided. In asking him how to move on from this, Ed himself suggested there was little merit in trying to resolve it with the anonymous faces of the organisation (and he had been gone about three months at this stage) and mentioned that his faith asked him to forgive. Sarah tentatively looked at this with him so that it was not an avoidance and then helped him reflect on what forgiveness would look like were he to entertain it as a possibility. She suggested a method that might help (Enright, 2001) based on research into the psychology of forgiveness. Ed thought this connected very well to his Christian faith and together they worked towards his letting go and forgiving those who he felt had wronged him.

Running this example briefly through the six steps of reflection helps us see the focus of each stage and the strategies that emerge from reflection at different levels. Different skills are needed at different stages, e.g., to move from Level 1 (zero reflection) to Level 2 (empathic reflection) needs the skill of empathy and emotional intelligence, the ability to see events from other perspectives. This can be taught and may need some practice to become fine-tuned. Moving from Level 2 to 3 and 4 requires being able to think relationally and systemically, to know how we set up systemic relationships where behaviour can be seen to be a result of those relationships. It also requires the skill of dialogue. Self-awareness skills, insights, awareness, openness and some courage is needed at Level 5 as we begin or continue the journey of insight into ourselves and our interpersonal and intrapersonal styles.

Level 6 is based on a belief of something beyond or further and often takes place when we are able to move beyond ourselves to principles that guide and support us. It would seem helpful to train or coach individuals and teams in the abilities needed to access all six levels of reflection.

A number of factors emerge while working with the six levels of reflection

First of all, while we started and moved through the levels systematically—from Level 1 to Level 6—it is not necessary to do so in that order. Many individuals go directly to Level 6, others move quickly to level 5 and ask: *"How am I contributing to this?"*. Reflection does not have to be sequential as presented here. Second, all levels of reflection are good. While levels sometimes gives the impression that the deeper I go the more valuable it is, the most helpful stance is being able to use all six levels as and when needed. There are times when I don't want to be empathic, dialogic, and negotiable and Level 1 is what is needed: *"That is not acceptable behaviour...I do not want to listen to you...You will need to change what you are doing"* is a valid response in some circumstances.

Each level of reflection brings valuable information pertinent to its own stage. At Levels 1 and 2, a supervisor can learn about how the other person (a supervisee) impacts on people in the outside world. Level 1 and 2 reflections give valuable information on the interpersonal world of the other (their interpersonal schema) and will also help you (as supervisor) see how you react to their interpersonal schema dependent on your own history (e.g., take up a persecutor, rescuer or a victim stance). Level 2 will give you an idea of how people can be empathic to others but still remain at a relationship distance—Level 3 is important for the reflector to achieve if they are to do good work with the other person. Level 4 gives good insights and information on the organisational and systemic contexts in which we work and sometimes ignore to our peril. Our own learning comes in Level 5 which we can feed back into Levels 3 and 4. It is important not to get fixated at stage 4 or 6 where we can over-reflect or become disconnected from the more grounded aspects of life.

As mentioned above, being able to move back and forth through all six levels (when appropriate) is the most mature response. Conversations or relationships are not helped when someone is stuck in one level and cannot reflect from within other levels. Difficulties arise when there are different levels of conversation and reflection in the same room, e.g., someone at Level 1 one can be certain of what they say and it will be difficult to have an open conversation if someone else is coming from Level 4. However, it is difficult to work with someone, as a coach or a supervisor, if I cannot allow myself or am unable to reflect in some of the areas they need to move into, e.g., some coaches would find it very difficult to allow religious belief into the coaching room since they themselves do not believe.

The skill of moving amongst these different levels of reflection is not just an individual competency but applies to couples, teams and organisations. It is legitimate to ask: At what level of reflection is this team? This organisation? Individuals, couples, teams and organisations have characteristic levels of reflection that they move towards automatically. Under stress they often revert to lower levels, e.g., Level 1.

These levels of reflection can be used in both life and work. Decision-making can rely on one level or another, or indeed on only one particular level. Ethics and religion can be seen from within each level and the types of ethics practiced (ethics of duty, ethics of trust, relational ethics, systemic ethics, etc.) can differ radically depending on which level is used to access it. There can also be blocks to reflection as we have indicated above, some particular to each level. Sometimes we need to ask at what level of reflection we need to be in order to resolve a particular problem we are facing. Perhaps problems don't get faced or resolved because we are not looking at them from an appropriate perspective, e.g., environmental issues and problems often need a systemic viewpoint and collaboration rather than simply an individualistic response.

There are also positive and negative stances at each level—see Table 4 below.

Level	Positive	Negative
1	Decisiveness, Non-negotiable Stances	Being Locked into one way of Seeing and Acting
2	Seeing Other Perspectives	Collusion with Others
3	Taking Relational Responsibility	Not Taking Personal Responsibility
4	Big Pictures	Missing Individuals
5	Increasing Self-awareness	Over Introspection
6	Deep Principles and Communal Values	Remoteness from Life and People

Table 4: Positive and Negative Stances at Each Level.

At times it may not be appropriate to use some levels, e.g., asking someone who has been bullied or harassed at work what contribution they made to being bullied (Level 5) would be very insensitive and could easily make them feel responsible for something outside their control.

These levels of reflection can be connected to different levels of learning (single loop learning, double and treble loop learning). As we move down the levels we move away from content (Levels 1 and 2) into process (Levels 3 and 4). Issues of how power is used (power over, power with, power through and power within) can also be applied to different levels, e.g., 'power over' is more of a Level 1 feature while 'power with' is more focused on Levels 3 and 4. 'Power within' can come with Levels 5 and 6. The movement through levels is not simply a cognitive one but a fully emotional one that involves the body as well as the mind (Carroll, 2009). Moore (2008) is working on reflective processes that involve enhanced and deepening self awareness, or what he calls 'emotional knowing' as part of supervision reflexivity. Individuals often reflect in and through their bodies. Consciousness raising takes place as we are able to access deeper levels (Kegan, 1994).

We ask what is the appropriate level of reflection to use with this person (coachee, supervisee) that best connects to where they are and challenges them to move towards their next level of learning?

Conclusion

For a long time we have presented 'reflective practice' as an ideal to be attained. Not only do we work, but through reflection on our work we learn how to do it better. However, there is little to help us learn how to reflect or to be able to deepen reflection. Here we make the point that access to all six levels of reflection creates the best environment for ongoing learning and suggests some methods to help move through the levels as appropriate.

Case example

How might you handle the following: *Bianca is a strong activist learner. She loves doing and is active in supervision in setting up role-plays to learn. She is not very good on reflection and tells you that when she stops to think her thoughts get all confused and she can make no sense of them. She is an excellent worker and you wonder whether or not you should help her be more reflective, even when it does not seem to suit her style.*

Have a look again at Appendices 16 (Reflection in Action: Questions for the Practitioner) which can help you reflect through the use of questions. Appendix 20 also contains a list of incisive questions to facilitate reflection.

Imagine yourself in supervision. You have a tricky situation you want to talk about. Think of an example of your work that has been difficult and caused you some concern. Now imagine your supervisor asking you to see this issue through the six positions of reflection. What would it be like for you to articulate the concern in these six different ways?

Review and Discussion

1. Can you describe what reflection means?
2. What are the deepening levels of reflection and could you say how a person might move to deeper levels?
3. How might you become more reflective?
4. What blocks reflection (your own, in particular) and how might you unblock it?
5. What do you think might happen in supervision if a supervisee was at a different (higher?) level of reflection than the supervisor?

CHAPTER 11

Supervisee Skill No. 4: Learning How to Give and Receive Feedback

Exercise

Before considering feedback, you might want to answer the following:

1. When someone says to you, *"I want to give you some feedback"*, what do you think? What do you feel? What do you do?

2. Do your reactions to giving (or receiving) feedback vary if delivered one-to-one versus feedback in a group?

3. Think back to your family of origin. Generally speaking, when you received feedback as a child, what did you feel?

4. After you have given someone feedback, have you ever wished that you had been more direct in what you said?

5. Complete this sentence: *"I feel more comfortable giving (or receiving) feedback when…"*

Do any of the following statements apply to you with respect to giving feedback?

1. I don't want to upset anyone or things. So best keep quiet.
2. If I wait long enough the situation will resolve itself.
3. It's not important enough to make a fuss over.
4. I don't want to increase distance between myself and the other person.
5. Criticising others reflects badly on me.
6. These are good people. They will know when they are getting things wrong.
7. I want others to take responsibility. Giving feedback takes that away.
8. I've made mistakes too so who am I to tell others what to do?
9. I find it very upsetting when I have to deliver strong negative feedback.
10. I told him twice and it hasn't made any difference, so why bother?
11. I don't know if I have enough evidence to confront him.
12. I could be wrong about this—perhaps she is right.
13. How can I criticise someone who is a friend? Good friends don't do that!
14. I feel really bad if I upset someone, and giving feedback upsets others at times.
15. I am afraid I might get angry if I really say what I want to say.
16. She has a very bitter tongue and I would come off worst if there were a fight.

17. I don't like receiving feedback myself so why should I impose it?

18. It will only embarrass both of us if I bring that up.

19. I don't like him anyway. I would be giving feedback for the wrong reasons.

Introduction to feedback

Of all the skills that supervisors and supervisees can possess, 'giving feedback' is perhaps the most sophisticated and difficult. We know some of the harmful results of receiving destructive feedback ('killer feedback', as someone once called it). Killer feedback hurts, wounds, shames and humiliates and does little to contribute to learning. Part of the problem with feedback is that we remember the feedback we received at the hands of others as children and it was frequently anything but positive. This is why people rarely ask for feedback, even to help their learning.

Otherwise we could regularly ask:

1. What is it like living with me?

2. What feedback would you like to give me as your parent, child, and manager?

3. What would you like to tell us about our being your employer?

These are dangerous questions. But why? You would think that we would ask for continual feedback in order to learn. Tell me...so that I can learn. But we are frightened we might hear what we fear most—I am no good, I should not be here, I am not worthwhile. We anticipate that all feedback will be negative and destructive because often that is the way it was in the past.

On the other hand, feedback connected to learning and feedback that is well-given and received is one of the best sources of learning for all of us. Think back to a moment when someone gave you valuable feedback that made a difference in your life. It probably was not easy to hear but when you heard it, it became a significant learning for you.

We want to learn, with you, how to give and receive feedback that is connected to learning.

Why feedback?

Feedback is necessary because there is much about ourselves that we do not know. We are often blind to the effects our behaviours have on others. We have blind spots (the 'baggage' that we carry from the past), hard spots (the assumptions that we have espoused from our training and 'believe' are facts) and 'dumb spots' (what we have yet to learn) (McLaughlin, 2005). Scharmer (2007) has a worthwhile grid that can help us name some of these 'spots':

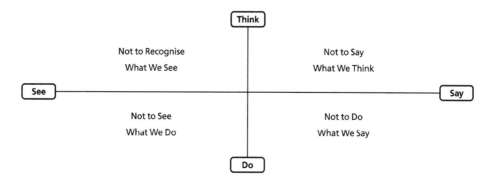

Figure 16: Feedback Grid (Scharmer, 2007)

There are things about ourselves we just don't know, either because we do not want to know (we are in denial) or because no one has ever told us and it is outside of our awareness. Knowing how you are perceived and experienced by others has always been important as a learning process. Knowledge about self in relation to others (how I relate to others, work with them, engage with them, talk to them, teach them, etc.) gives us the insights we need to help us begin to change our behaviours. Such knowledge is vital for the effective working of teams and organisations.

It is a well-established psychological principle that we judge ourselves by our intentions and we judge others by their behaviour. Our own feedback to ourselves comes from an internal awareness of what our intentions are: on the other hand we go 'external' in our evaluations of the behaviours of others. We judge what we see. Hence the discrepancy in how we and others see the same behaviour. The racist says: *"I am no racist"* (and from an intentionality perspective that is true—in their own minds their intention is to 'tell the truth as they see it'). I do not see their intentions, I see their behaviour and we define racism by what we do (not by what we intend). I see the discrimination, the prejudice at work and the words that are part of the truth. This is one of the reasons why feedback is so important: it helps all of us who focus on our intentions to hear another perspective—that of the outsider.

Example

Nigel is unaware that he gets frustrated and angry when his challenges in the group do not work as effectively as he hopes. When he challenges and the recipient does not respond as he had expected, he becomes impatient and ends up bullying. As we watched the video together, I asked him about his intentions regarding Alan, a member of the group. "I want to challenge him to look at his aggressive behaviour, and so I confront him with the inconsistencies between what he says and what he does", replies Nigel. "What happens then?", I probe. "I challenge him clearly and firmly," says Nigel, "but when he ignores me I go after him". I then give him feedback on what I see, namely that he begins to challenge well but the challenge descends into harassment when he loses his patience and cannot stay with the pace of the participant in the group. Nigel responds with interest, "You're right, I wanted to challenge and ended up harassing; what I need to watch is how impatient I get and how often I do not go at the other person's pace."

Clearly, Nigel does not deny what is happening and is using feedback to learn about himself, his style and his way of interaction. Pat, on the other hand, denies what is going on.

"How dare you tell me my presentation skills are only average? I have been doing this for four years now and no one has ever said that to me".

What is feedback?

Feedback is information on behaviour (observable behaviours are the focus) and the effects that behaviour has on others. Rock (2006) put it well when he describes feedback as *'...the delicate art of letting people know the score. Feedback gives people information that helps them learn and grow'* (p. 203). It can be either confirmatory (want more of it) or corrective (want less of it) or reflective (hold it up to the light to review it). The purpose of feedback is to facilitate learning and help change behaviour. This is why, in giving feedback, people need to be aware of their own motivation. If you are giving feedback for reasons other than to help the other person learn, then this invalidates the purpose of feedback. Clear, brief sentences based on observable behaviour (without using qualifiers) are best. And its purpose is to help the recipient *learn*, not to put them down, deskill, humiliate or demotivate them. However, we have already looked at what impacts negatively on our learning. Rock (2006) summarises this, *'When we experience anxiety, fear, self-consciousness or any strong emotion, our neurons get flooded with electrical signals, so there's not enough capacity left to process what is going on in the moment. We literally stop hearing and seeing what's around us'* (p. 61). It is worth remembering that if feedback is to be effective (as a learning format) then it has to be given within a relationship and an environment that does not cause the above reactions.

Feedback consists of the following:

1. The *what* of feedback (what do I want to say?).
2. The *how* of feedback (how do I do it?).
3. The *emotions* of feedback (emotional barriers are the main obstacles inhibiting the exchange of feedback).

4. The *when* of feedback (the right moment).
5. The *where* of feedback (the right place).

Exercise

Take an example of someone (in the past) that you would have liked to have given feedback to and see if you can use the features above to formulate how you might say it to them.

Exercise

Feedback to self on Feedback. What helps and hinders me from giving and receiving feedback?

	Giving Feedback	Receiving Feedback
Helps		
Hinders		

Figure 17: Feedback to Self on Feedback

Some of the elements that we need to consider when giving and receiving feedback are:

1. Our own background and learning: strong cultural and family backgrounds encourage us to be nice to people and not say things that make them uncomfortable. 'Don't cause conflict' is often a dictate we inherit from the past.
2. We sometimes equate feedback with criticism. There is some evidence to indicate that childhood feedback was painful for most people and the existence of a link between past negative experiences of feedback and the ability to do it now. Think back to your experience of receiving feedback as a child—what was it like?

3. Our difficulty with causing conflict. Is this a problem for you?

4. How will the other person interpret it: will they feel or be hurt? Are you anxious about the person receiving feedback?

5. Difficulty of self esteem; we are sometimes worried that if we give negative feedback we will damage the positive self-image or the self-esteem of the person to whom we give this feedback.

6. We know that feedback is often connected not just to our behaviour but to how we see ourselves as persons. At times this connects with our fear that we are no good and not worth loving.

7. We think, at times, that we have no permission to comment on the behaviour and skills of another person.

Giving and receiving feedback

In giving feedback (and receiving it) it is worth reminding ourselves of what is helpful or not helpful:

Helpful	Unhelpful
Descriptive	Evaluative
Specific	General
Two-sided	One-sided
Solicited	Unsolicited
Current	Historic
Relevant	Irrelevant
Offered	Imposed
Checked	Unchecked
Recognises Emotion	Ignores Emotion
Open	Closed
Direct	Indirect

Figure 18: Giving and Receiving Feedback

Exercise

Go back to the exercise above where you were giving feedback to someone from your past and run it through the above characteristics.

A key to effective feedback is to understand the other in terms of:

1. His/her way of learning: emotional, intellectual, etc.

2. How much time do they need to talk through, to hear?

3. Ability to hear undefensively (how defended are they?).
4. How able are they to be in touch with themselves?
5. How am I perceived and experienced by the other person?

Occasionally, when feedback goes wrong, we can trace it to the following:

1. Burying the message so that it is unclear.
2. Playing the psychologist and interpreting the inner meaning of what is going on.
3. Questioning can become interrogation.
4. Softening, disclaiming or apologising for the feedback.
5. Agreement that is not real agreement.
6. Going on and on without stopping to check in or listen back.

Reactions of the receiver:

1. Playing the wounded animal (hurt, devastated, wounded, exaggerated).
2. Changing the subject.
3. Attacking as the best form of defense.
4. Using comparisons with others (lobbying).
5. Becoming the masochist and inviting more negative feedback (punish me more!).

Steps to giving feedback:

1. How can I create the most conducive environment for the person to receive the feedback I intend on giving?
2. How do I ensure an open rapport and free interchange?
3. Is the person ready to hear what I want to say?
4. What would stop me giving feedback just now?
5. How am I feeling about giving feedback just now?
6. Am I open to changing my views in the light of the discussion?
7. Am I clear about what I want to share?
8. Am I giving this feedback from a place of goodwill, i.e., to help learning?

Giving feedback itself: How can I…

1. Bring about an open rapport and a free interchange?
2. Know whether the person is ready and in what state of mind?
3. Keep comments close to the events described?

4. Ensure agreement?

5. Keep in touch with what is happening to me?

6. Be open to changing my own opinion?

7. Know when it might be helpful to refrain from giving feedback?

8. Be aware of the emotional barriers that can make giving and receiving feedback very difficult?

9. Make sure that feedback is not just positive and/or negative: it is well-rounded feedback on how someone is doing?

10. Check that what I intended to say was heard?

11. Identify the areas that need improvement/change?

12. Identify how that improvement or change will take place?

After giving feedback:

1. Spend a little time reviewing the meeting. Is there something to be filed away for the next meeting?

2. What did I learn about myself?

3. What did I learn about the other person?

4. What did I learn about giving feedback?

Exercise

The following is a short exercise to help you prepare for receiving feedback and be open to learning during a feedback session.

Receiving feedback:

Preparing myself to listen:

1. Am I anxious about what another person might say?

2. What would stop me from listening?

3. Am I feeling defensive? Attacked?

4. How do I feel about the person who is giving me feedback?

5. Am I open to what others will say?

Before the feedback session, ask yourself:

1. Do I want to learn from this session?

2. Am I open to what the other person is going to say?

3. Do I want to consider how what is said can help me develop either personally and/or professionally?

4. Am I in the right frame of mind to engage with this feedback?

5. Is this feedback about my behaviour?

Listen carefully to what is said by the person or persons giving you feedback:

1. Articulate feelings, especially if you or the other are finding it difficult to hear the feedback being given.

2. Summarise what is said so that we are agreed on the content.

3. Ask for clarification, if needed, or specifics or examples.

4. Own the feedback (make it yours) fully or partially. Or, after considering it, disagree with it. Discuss it.

5. Begin to dialogue about how the feedback can be used to help you change.

6. Agree what needs to be done, with whose help, by what date.

7. End feedback session.

The Theory of Core Qualities (Ofman, 2001)

The *Theory of Core Qualities* is a model devised for HR managers on how to give negative feedback in a positive and constructive manner. Have a look and see if you can use it in your supervision to find areas you need to work on for yourself or indeed to give feedback to self and others.

The model suggests (see Figure 22) four interconnected positions leading to a quadrant. The four are:

1. *Core Qualities* are attributes that form part of a person's core. Those who know the individual will recognise the qualities immediately. Core qualities are positive and are the strengths of an individual and mostly present in their lives. Examples of core qualities are: determination, loyalty, empathy, hard working, courage, humility, flexibility, etc. Core qualities are recognised by what others appreciate in me, what I expect/demand from others and often what I play down in myself.

2. *Pitfalls* exist when an individual exercises too much of their core quality. The Pitfall is an overdeveloped core quality. It is the area where most of us get negative feedback. You can recognise areas for your Pitfall by what you are willing to forgive in others, what others blame you for (negative feedback) and often by what you try to justify in yourself. The philosophy behind this is that our weaknesses are not the opposites of our strengths but rather too much of our actual strength:

   A. Determination becomes pushiness or control when taken too far.

    B.   Loyalty becomes collusion.

    C.   Empathy becomes enmeshment.

    D.   Helpfulness becomes interference.

3.   *The Challenge* is the direct opposite of the Pitfall and combined with the Core Quality keeps individuals out of the Pitfall. You will know your challenges by what you miss in yourself, what you admire in others and what others want for you.

    A.   Determination needs patience to not end up as pushiness.

    B.   Flexibility needs orderliness to not become inconsistency.

    C.   Loyalty needs objectivity or questioning to not end up as collusion.

4.   *The Allergy* is a reaction to too much of our challenge and the opposite of the Core Quality. It is what I cannot stand in myself and in others. You will know it by what you despise in others, what I would hate in myself.

Example

Let us run an example through the Theory of Core Qualities. One of us (Michael) is the executive coach to a Project Manager (Jeremy) in a large company. Jeremy phones up unexpectedly to make an appointment, very upset by an event that has happened in his workplace. On arrival he launches into his story about being labelled 'a bully' or 'someone who harasses'. This has upset him greatly as he has never envisaged himself as such. Briefly, the event happened during a meeting with one of his staff, a new graduate who is working with him on a particular project. Three hours into their meeting she suddenly puts her head in her hands and shouts at him: *"Leave me alone, I cannot take any more. I feel bullied by you. This is not the first time you have harassed me"*. He ends the meeting and arranges his executive coaching session.

We put 'bullying and harassment' into the Pitfall and I ask him what was he doing too much of to have it labelled 'bullying or harassment'. He knew immediately, *"I was being action-oriented"*, he said. So, I summarised, *"If action-oriented was your core quality and bullying or harassment is your Pitfall, what is your Challenge"*? Again he knew almost immediately. *"Going at her pace"*. And of course, his Allergy is individuals who never get things done (no action). We now plan for the future and I coach him in how to stay action-oriented and proceed at the pace of the slowest member to ensure the individual and the team is with him. He saw the sense: the poor member of staff was exhausted, had no break for nearly three hours and felt compelled to remain engaged when she needed to get away. For Jeremy not to end up in his Pitfall he had to learn how to go at the speed of others and to not just engage with his own high levels of stamina and energy.

It would have been easy for me (his coach) to lecture him on the ills of bullying or harassment but the Theory of Core Qualities gave him an understanding and insight into this behaviour that does not just concentrate on the negative. It places the negative (the Pitfall) in a much larger picture where the weaknesses are seen as related to the strengths. This does not justify what happens in the Pitfall but it makes it more easily understood and accepted when placed in the wider context.

1. Decisive people (core quality) will be allergic to passiveness.
2. Empathic people (core quality) will have an allergy to selfishness.
3. Loyal individuals will be allergic to betrayal or deceit.

In brief the model looks like this:

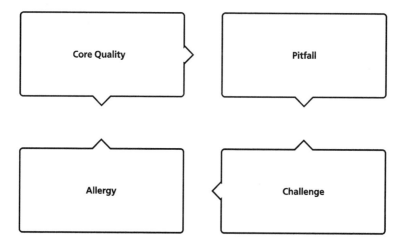

Figure 19: Theory of Core Qualities

1. The Pitfall is too much of the Core Quality.
2. The Challenge is the positive opposite of the Pitfall.
3. The Allergy is too much of the challenge.
4. The Core Quality is the positive opposite of the Allergy.

Exercise

Go to Appendix 13 and see if you can fill in the four areas of the quadrant for yourself.

Conclusion

Giving and receiving feedback are both demanding processes. They take some courage and a good deal of skill. The focus of feedback (negative or positive) is to facilitate learning. The best learning is a process of practice, feedback, practice, feedback, practice, feedback, etc.

Case example

If you were the supervisor, how might you work with Jane to help her be less controlling and be open to feedback?

Jane always arrived at supervision very well prepared with typed notes regarding the client she wished to present and a list of three questions she wished to focus upon in supervision. On the face of it she was an exemplary supervisee since she was always well prepared. She might start by saying: "I will give you a brief summary of the last session and then I would like you to focus on the questions I have brought". In this way she controlled her supervision group and ensured that no one asked any 'uncomfortable' questions. It was only when Jane agreed to bring an audio-taped session with a client and start playing it at a random place that the supervisor was able to give her feedback on her actual work. She found the feedback, some of which was negative, very difficult to hear and accept. When they examined the situation in more detail, Jane agreed with the supervisor that in fact she had previously thought of all the answers to the questions on her list so supervision seldom yielded anything new/surprising or actually helpful to her! She realised that shameful experiences in her childhood family and subsequently at school had led her to 'protect' herself in this way.

Review and discussion

1. Are you clear about how feedback is connected to learning?
2. Can you see the connections between how we give and receive feedback now and our past history of giving and receiving feedback?
3. Do you have a clear method and approach to giving feedback that helps another person learn (a framework)?
4. Can you now be open and free to listen to feedback (especially critical or negative feedback) as a way of learning?

Appendix 2 and 3 have evaluation forms for a supervision session and for giving feedback to your supervisor. Fill out both of these now.

CHAPTER 12

Supervisee Skill No 5: Learning Realistic Self-evaluation

Evaluation refers to the process of assessing the competence of our work in terms of its effectiveness and the desired outcomes. Clearly, this is a central aspect of supervision. As we mentioned in our discussion on developmental stages in the learning process, the aim of professional learning is to develop a reliable 'internal supervisor' (Casement,1985) who can evaluate our own competence as we go along. Carroll (1996) separates out the *'evaluating'* and the *'monitoring'* tasks of supervision. Evaluation includes the provision of ongoing feedback in supervision sessions and the overall evaluation of your work at certain points. In training contexts this occurs usually at the end of the academic year, and again, and most significantly, at the point of qualification. We see evaluation as an ongoing process in supervision that, at its best, is a collaborative process with clearly agreed goals and milestones that are defined and stipulated along the way.

One of the biggest challenges for any professional is learning realistic self-evaluation. Most of the people we meet in supervision are very hard on themselves and tend to criticise all they do in a negative and disqualifying manner. This is doubly difficult because: a) they do not recognise what they do effectively and where their realistic points of development may be; and b) they also tend to overreact to any suggestions made by the supervisor that they may interpret as a complete negation of themselves. If you get into a process of this kind, it will be very difficult for anyone to give you anything useful! The secret is to develop the capacity to receive feedback, listen to it carefully, evaluate it for yourself and use it as the basis for further learning and setting further learning goals.

The aim of supervision is for the supervisee to develop an internal supervisor that is well-balanced, well-informed and realistic about goal setting. What is important is to be very clear about the goals or outcomes you want to achieve and then look at the criteria by which you will assess these.

Specific criteria will, of course, be related to your particular area of work but it may be helpful to look at some general guidelines here.

1. What is your goal or aim in this piece of work?
2. How will you know that you have achieved a successful outcome?
3. What specific behavioural criteria will you use to assess your performance?

4. What do you most appreciate about what you did?

5. What would you do differently next time?

6. What have you learned from this particular analysis?

7. What is your next area for development?

Self-evaluation can involve different areas. Gilbert and Sills (1999) describe three 'lenses' through which evaluation can take place: a) a focus on micro-skills; b) a focus on a particular session or task; and c) a focus on development over time. We will discuss each of these in turn to show how they can enhance and build realistic self-evaluation of work.

Micro-skills

This involves an interaction-by-interaction analysis of a session or segment of a session (or a group session or a meeting) with a view to identifying effective and non-effective interventions and practicing alternatives. An audio or video recording is of particular help in this micro-analytic process.

Exercise

Choose an intervention that you considered effective and reflect on this in terms of the client's immediate (and subsequent) responses. How can you tell (by change of energy, intensity of affect, etc.) that you have 'reached' this client?

Exercise

Choose a point in the work where you were particularly aware that you had a choice and could have made a number of different responses/interventions. Focus on the choice point and recall what you were thinking at that time.

1. What other options were you considering?

2. What led you to make this particular choice (for example, client considerations, contextual factors, diagnostic considerations)? What made you feel it may be the best way forward or did you make it because you were scared of conflict and therefore chose the line of least resistance?

3. Do you consider that your choice led to an effective outcome? If so, why? If not, why?

4. How does the choice of this particular intervention relate to your theoretical orientation?

5. What might you wish to experiment with differently in the future? Practice a few alternatives. (Gilbert & Evans, 2000, p. 52).

Role-play is a useful way to practise alternative interventions particularly if you are in group supervision and another member can role-play the client. In this way you can experiment with new options and get immediate feedback from others about the effectiveness of your interventions. You can begin to widen your repertoire of micro-skills and get immediate feedback to evaluate your new points of learning. Such exposure to the feedback of others is helpful in developing realistic self-evaluation and can help us to begin to 'see ourselves as others see us' rather than hanging on to unrealistic self-assessments.

Evaluation of a session or a task

Here the evaluation will relate to a completed session or task. Again you will first be looking at whether you have achieved your overall goal or aim in this piece of work. As an example of a sessional evaluation, we will provide some questions to consider that could arise in a supervision session.

1. Did you and the supervisor mutually agree on a clear and manageable contract for the session?
2. In other words, did you negotiate specific objectives, and explicit and measurable goals?
3. Was this contract completed by the end of the session?
4. Did you clarify your expectations for the session?
5. Did the session allow for an honest and open exchange?
6. Did the supervisor provide both support and confrontation?
7. Was feedback specific, respectful and related to the contract?
8. Did the session provide a balance of action and reflection?
9. Was the atmosphere warm and collaborative?
10. Did you experiment with new options/ideas with the support of the supervisor?
11. Did you have fun in the learning process?

(Gilbert & Sills, 1999).

These questions are based on some of the findings from outcome research on supervision that highlights the qualities inherent in effective supervision. You can draw up a similar list for any task in terms of the standards for that piece of work and then use these criteria as a guideline for realistic self-evaluation. Vagueness about the criteria we use for self-assessment can encourage falling back into self-criticism and self-depreciating comments that have little basis in the reality of our efforts. The question remains: What are the specific criteria by which we are evaluating our performance? And are these realistic and achievable?

Here is a short supervision checklist from Gilbert and Sills (1999) that will help you review a supervision session quickly:

1. What was your contract and have you met it?
2. What have you found most useful from your supervisor?
3. What do you want more of from your supervisor?
4. What do you want less of from your supervisor?
5. What is the next developmental edge for you?

Evaluating development over time

Sometimes, in supervision, we wish to review our development over the past year or our progress in a particular job over a specified period of time. This means taking a longer view of aims and goals and achievements (and of goals not realised). Such a review will involve a discussion of particular goals related to your performance but will also include questions about your overall satisfaction in the job. Some questions that might help you reflect on your motivation are:

1. Do I enjoy what I am doing?
2. What is my primary motivation for doing this work?
3. Does my job give me satisfaction?
4. Am I learning what I need to support myself well?
5. Have I made a choice of career that suits my abilities and proclivities?
6. What am I most passionate about in this area of work?

Supervisees are well advised to agree to learning goals with the supervisor for a period of time—usually for the next year—so that they have an overall learning plan. Such goals may be: to focus on the integration of theory into practice; to broaden and increase their repertoire of skills; to firm up on assessment skills; to hone my presentation skills; to improve the clarity of my problem formulations, etc. In this way, as a supervisee, you will not only have a contract for a particular session but will also have an overall learning goal for the year that relates to your ongoing development as a professional. These longer-term goals could be reviewed every three months to assess your progress and focus anew on your growing edges as a practitioner. These longer-term contracts can also cover new areas that you wish to be introduced to by your supervisor and to receive guidance in developing and exploring.

Supervision contracts are often made for a year at a time so the last session of each year's supervision contract could be used to review this level of your learning and development with a view to looking forward to the next phase. Sometimes this may involve moving on to another supervisor with a different orientation or skills area so that you can get new challenges.

Conclusion

Our hope in this section is that you will be able to evaluate yourself and your competencies realistically, without being too positive or too negative on yourself. Self-evaluation is a key to progress. Combined with supervisor evaluation, and the evaluations of significant others, it becomes a marvellous tool for learning.

Case example

How might you deal with the supervisee in this instance?

Jack always presents in supervision very positively and never brings any of his work that is negative. You are not sure if he does not feel safe enough to share his vulnerability or if he has an inflated sense of his own work. You suspect the latter, i.e., that he is not able to make a balanced and realistic evaluation of his work. You are wondering how to talk to him to help him be more real about his achievements and abilities without devastating him.

Review and discussion

1. Do you consider yourself able to be realistic about evaluating yourself and your work? Is your tendency to be more positive than negative, or vice-versa?

2. Do you have clear criteria against which you evaluate yourself professionally?

3. Can you see the beginnings of 'an internal supervisor' that monitors your work while you are doing it and evaluates what you are doing realistically?

4. Can you see how your evaluation of yourself can be set within a developmental process—where you have come from and where you are going?

CHAPTER 13

Supervisee Skill No 6: Learning Emotional Awareness

Emotions are often the forgotten side of supervision and learning. Supervision is an emotional experience and how we deal with the emotional side of supervision relationships, of feedback in supervision, of assessment, evaluation and supervision reports—not to mention disputes, conflicts and disagreement—is often not even considered on the supervision agenda. Weisinger (1998) writes about *'emotional fallout'* when feedback is delivered destructively. Emotional intelligence helps us deal with many of these supervisory issues.

In general, women are more emotionally aware than men (Orme, 2001). So men, in particular, have to pay attention to their ability to tune into feelings—their own and those of others—and take appropriate action. We know also that feelings and the ability to express them is connected to upbringing (e.g., big boys don't cry), can be connected to culture and race (some cultures are more accepting of expressing feelings, e.g., the British have a reputation of having a 'stiff upper lip').

Emotional Intelligence

Goleman (1996), in his now famous book *'Emotional Intelligence'*, defines it as the *'capacity for recognising our feelings and those of others, for motivating ourselves and for managing emotions well in ourselves and in our relationships'*. Feelings help us stay in touch with ourselves and our values. They help us make decisions and facilitate us moving on (the word emotion is derived from the Latin verb *'to move'*). Emotional language allows us to put our feelings into words and hence be able to deal with them more effectively and constructively. Weisinger (1998) suggests four building blocks to emotional literacy:

1. The ability to perceive, appraise and express emotion accurately.
2. The ability to access or generate feelings on demand when they can facilitate understanding of yourself or another person.
3. The ability to understand emotions and the knowledge that derives from them.
4. The ability to regulate emotions.

Ways of managing emotions

Individuals have different ways to handle and manage their feelings. Some of these are:

1. Being aware of feelings and expressing them appropriately.
2. Not being in touch with feelings—they come out in other ways rather than appropriate expression (e.g., I kick the dog rather than get angry with my father).
3. Engulfed with feelings (e.g., road rage, violence, etc.).
4. Somatise emotions (they come out in physical reactions—pain in the body, headaches, etc.).

Carl Rogers (2004) talked about seven levels of feelings:

1. Not owned, not recognised, not in touch with.
2. Owned, but talked about as in the past.
3. Feelings are described rather than felt.
4. Feelings are owned but externalised (well, one would feel angry).
5. Feelings are expressed as present.
6. There is a flow of feelings.
7. Access to full feelings as they happen and ability to express them appropriately.

Exercise

Use Rogers' *Seven Levels of Feelings* to see where you are with regard to owning and expressing certain feelings. Look at the list in Appendix 11 to help you.

Exercise

How in touch are you with your feelings?
See Goleman's *Emotional Competency Framework* outlined in Appendix 10.

Here are some processes that might help you to get in touch with feelings and be able to act appropriately on them:

1. Recognise the importance of feelings.
2. Give feelings permission to be.
3. Acknowledge feelings.
4. Realise there are no good or bad feelings—feelings are feelings.

5. Listen to and observe your body—it might let you know about feelings.

6. Every so often stop and finish the sentence, *"Just now, I am feeling…"*.

7. Listen to your feelings—what are they saying to you?

8. Listen to the feelings of other people—ask yourself, what is this person feeling now?

9. Put another person's feelings into words (not necessarily for them but for yourself), e.g., *"This person is feeling…"*.

10. Are there some feelings you are more comfortable with than others. Some people deny certain feelings, *"Am I am feeling…hurt…or anger…or fear?"*.

11. Can you distinguish within feelings? For example, there is a continuum from mild irritation to fury with feelings such as anger somewhere along the continuum.

12. Can you distinguish between feelings such as hurt, resentment, anger, sadness? Some people get feelings mixed up with regard to intensity or duration.

13. Distinguish between thoughts, feelings and actions.

14. Can you take time between feeling and doing? Some people are very impulsive with feelings and do not take a measured response which, at times, can help.

15. Begin to monitor how your body reacts to certain feelings (e.g., *"I feel scared—there are butterflies in my stomach, my mouth dries up, I cannot focus, my palms are sweaty."*).

16. Have a look at a list of feeling words (see Appendix 11). Which feelings do you find easy to acknowledge and express, which ones are difficult for you to accept and articulate appropriately?

17. Are there some feelings you 'privatise', i.e., you pull them inside yourself and do not express them in an appropriate way, e.g., some people do this with anger (once privatised it can then become depression).

18. Have a look at layers of feelings (guilt and shame can come together, or anger and hurt and guilt all get mingled).

19. Sometimes we have to deal with a backlog of feelings, i.e., feelings that have remained unexpressed for some time, e.g., loss and bereavement can be triggered by a present event (we lay what someone referred to as *'gunpowder trails'* where an occurrence in the present can trigger an explosion from the past).

Ostell, Baverstock and Wright (1999) suggest some principles for managing emotions that are helpful for supervisees:

Principle 1: Deal with the emotional reaction before attempting to resolve the problem.

1. Engage the rational when the level of emotion is reduced.
2. Reflective statements are very helpful.
3. Apologise if appropriate.
4. Acknowledge the feeling.
5. Stay with it as long as is needed.

Principle 2: Avoid behaviours that heighten adverse emotional reactions.

1. Some reactions heighten the emotion rather than reduce it, e.g., words such as stupid, worthless, etc.
2. Unconstructive mood matching (e.g., anger for anger, sarcasm for sarcasm). I respond in the same mood as you.
3. A type of confrontation that simply disparages another's emotional experience, e.g., *"Don't be childish, grow up, getting upset won't help"*.

Principle 3: Employ behaviours likely to dissipate adverse emotional reactions.

1. Empathy to indicate understanding.
2. Giving permission to express emotion.
3. Normalising the emotion, e.g., *"It's ok to feel that way"*.
4. 'Time out' to recompose and continue at a later date.
5. Give ideas that might help resolve the issues.
6. Empathise with the person.

Principle 4: Recognise differences between emotions.

Different emotions tend to be provoked and sustained by different ways of thinking, e.g., three employees who have failed to get a promotion:

1. One feels angry: violation of rights (*"I should have been…"*).
2. One feels anxious: anticipates negative consequences (*"I'm stuck here."*).
3. One feels depressed: helplessness and self-blame (*"It's my fault."*).

Some suggested responses:

1. To the angry—apologise.
2. Anxious—the consequences are manageable and may not be so bad.

3. Depressed—getting some control and power.

The more deeply these emotions are felt the more professional the help required.

Principle 5: Where appropriate, attempt to find a solution to the underlying problem.

1. Unless the underlying problem is dealt with, the negative emotional response is likely to re-occur.
2. It may be enough to have emotional expression and understanding.
3. Non-directive approach: helping another find the solution.
4. Directive methods: giving advice, problem solving.

Principle 6: Learn to accept reality actively.

1. Some situations cannot be solved (e.g., loss and death).
2. Some cannot be resolved because of others (redundancy, neighbours, etc.).

Managers use the following in managing emotions at work:

1. Deal with disruptive emotional behaviour.
2. Learn the importance of distinguishing between everyday emotional reaction (reactions to missed deadlines, bonus at work, etc.) and emotional problems of a more complicated nature (PTSD, chronic depression, paranoia).
3. Help staff find ways to better manage situations and their reactions instead of trying to diagnose problems.
4. Refer for expert help when necessary.

Conclusion

Learning 'emotional literacy' will help you deal more effectively with the kinds of issues that arise in your work and in your supervision. Emotions are not just internal reactions but connect us—in ways we sometimes cannot even imagine—to life and others. Far from being simply distraction to tolerate or accept passively, feelings become the 'inner rudder' of our lives, personally and professionally.

Case example

How might you work with Fred?

To put it mildly, Fred is emotionally illiterate—he is not in touch with his own feelings and rarely acknowledges the feelings of others. You have seen him, on a number of occasions, ignore deep feelings of anger and loss in his group and in the individuals with whom he works. When asked how he feels, he moves straight into thoughts. You are wondering what you can do to help him get in touch with his feelings and the feelings of others that, in your view, would make him a much better worker.

Review and discussion

1. What is the importance of being aware of emotions within supervision?
2. How emotionally aware are you? What areas need development?
3. How can one become more emotionally aware?

CHAPTER 14

Supervisee Skill No 7: Learning How to Dialogue

Supervision is a conversation, a talk that centres on the work of the supervisee. Like all conversations it can take on many forms:

1. A monologue where one person is speaking (e.g., if the supervisor is giving an overview on how to work with a certain kind of client group).

2. A negotiation (where the supervision contract is being devised).

3. A discussion where a number of people share ideas on a subject (e.g., sharing ideas on how to approach a particular problem that a supervisee has brought to a supervision group).

4. A debate where there is usually a win/lose segment (looking at the pros and cons of a counselling orientation).

5. An argument where one person is trying to convince the other about the rightness of their position (where a supervisee is trying to persuade the supervisor that her interventions were appropriate to the situation).

While all these modes of conversation have their place in supervision and can be helpful methods of learning, the best overall method of supervisory conversation is dialogue.

What is dialogue?

'Dialogue means a flow of meaning. It is a conversation in which we think together in relationship' (Isaacs, 1999).

'Dialogue is the encounter of those addressed to the common task of learning and acting' (Freire, 1998, p. 74).

'Dialogue is talk—a special kind of talk—that affirms the person-to-person relationship between discussants and which acknowledges their collective right and intellectual capacity to make sense of the world' (Dixon, 1998, p. 59).

Exercise

Look and select some conversation on TV and see if you can decide what kind of talk is taking place: is it a discussion, a monologue, a debate, an argument?

1. What are the features of these different kinds of conversations?

Features of dialogue

The features that distinguish dialogue from other forms of conversation include the following:

1. It is based on a certain kind of relationship. Dixon (1998) writes: *'I am suggesting that dialogue is not a difference in technique, but a difference in relationship'* (p. 63). The relationship is one of valuing, respect, and equality. Dialogue is a meeting of people who come together to learn from each other.

2. It is a certain stance of humility towards learning. Knowing I do not know all there is to know allows me to come to others with openness to learning.

3. Dialogue acknowledges that we each see the world from a certain perspective (psychological truth) and that for each of us, there are other legitimate perspectives.

4. Dialogue does not have a pre-existing outcome—those taking part are never certain where the conversation might go. Dialogue therefore means being open to various outcomes—the way forward.

Isaacs (1999) outlines four features of dialogue:

1. The ability to listen (to myself, to others, to other perspectives).
2. The ability to respect (others, their views).
3. The ability to suspend (my own certainty, my own truth).
4. The ability to voice (to articulate, to say, to allow and help others to voice their thoughts and feelings).

The idea of play has been applied to supervision (Hawkins & Shohet, 2000). This is not to trivialise work or the people with whom one works, but to bring a curious and inquiring attitude to work that allows us to consider other ways of thinking about it. In a sense this is what dialogue does too. It plays with thoughts, ideas, stories, other perspectives, viewpoints, opinions, intuitions, hunches, theories, and frameworks as ways to approach helpful actions. *'Generative learning'* or *'generative dialogues'* are terms used to show how talk leads to action.

Multicultural aspects of the supervisory process

Conversations are between people and people differ in an amazing number of ways. These differences can too easily become ways to divide us or, in dialogue, hopefully enrich us.

How would you name difference in supervision and keep open your awareness of individual differences that impact on your relationships? We need to keep open our awareness of how issues of difference may impact on our work: issues of race, disability, age, gender, sexual orientation, religion, politics, language, culture and ethnicity. When we are working with a person from a different culture, we will need to take care to enquire into the 'norms' of that culture and take care not to assume they are the same as ours. In general, it is easy to do this in relation to the most obvious behavioural cues (dress, eating habits, etc.), but it is not as easy in relation to more embedded beliefs and assumptions about life and work (those that we likely take for granted or value without thinking).

Some useful questions to ask of ourselves in supervision:

1. How may this person be seeing me?
2. What do I bring to this relationship in terms of my background that may subtly influence the relationship?
3. How aware am I of the impact of my behaviour, assumptions and attitudes on other people I have worked with? What can I learn from my experience of my impact on others?
4. How may the political context in which I am functioning influence the relationship?
5. What do I need to know about the race/culture/sexual orientation, etc., of this person in order to help him/her effectively or to have a good working relationship?
6. What reading can I do that will help me to understand differences?
7. Can I imaginatively put myself into the 'shoes' of the other person and begin to get a sense of how he/she experiences her world?
8. What prejudices do I have that may hamper our relationship? Am I willing to be honest with myself about these and work to eradicate them?
9. If you are working in a culture that is not your own, what steps have you taken to get to know the norms and assumptions of your host culture?
10. What assumptions are you bringing from your culture of origin that would be viewed as eccentric at best, or pathological and dangerous at worst?

Conclusion

Supervision is a form of conversation closer to dialogue than to any other form of talk. In dialogue, both parties (supervisees and supervisors) work together towards conclusions and solutions. These do not necessarily pre-exist and in the openness, discussion and honesty of supervision, the best way forward emerges. Like so many other areas of supervision it is here, in the conversation we call supervision, that issues of *power* emerge—such issues have to be dealt with openly (through dialogue) so that power is used to empower rather than disempower.

Case example

Any suggestions for how to work with Alison:

Alison is always right. She finds it hard to listen to other points of view in supervision. Her thinking is rigid and when she makes up her mind it is very difficult to get her to rethink her conclusions. As a result, you get lots of monologues from her. She has recently converted to being a born-again Christian and has begun to lecture the small supervision group on how important it is for them to have faith and belief in God and Jesus. You can see it is having a negative effect on participants in the group.

Review and discussion

1. What are the differences between monologue, discussion, debate, argument and dialogue?
2. What are the characteristics of dialogue?
3. How do we set up the environment and relationships that allow dialogue to occur?
4. What do you see as the difficulties in your situation that would make dialogue difficult to attain?

CHAPTER 15

Using the Supervision Group

Supervision in groups is a common format in many professions. Groups provide a rich source of learning since you have the group members to draw from in addition to the supervisor.

Advantages of group supervision

1. You can hear about the work of other group members, which may be very different from your own, and can gain knowledge by proxy.

2. Sometimes another group member will present an issue similar to one you are dealing with and this will be of direct help to you.

3. You will get a sense of what your peers are struggling with and this provides a sense of twin-ship with others that can be reassuring.

4. Interacting with others in a professional group like this where open communication is fostered provides a good model to draw upon in respective work contexts.

5. Other group members may have knowledge and experience that you, the supervisor or the rest of the group members do not possess and this can provide a rich source of collegial sharing.

6. In a well-functioning group, there is the benefit of learning 'in vivo' from the process in the group about those factors that contribute to a healthy learning environment for you and others.

Potential hazards in group supervision

1. Competitiveness for the attention of the supervisor, or competition about time and who gets how much, may jeopardise the effectiveness of the group.

2. One member may end up dominating the group and unless this is confronted early on, could lead to dissatisfaction or even the dissolution of the group.

3. Group members may not voice their expectations clearly or deal openly with conflicts and disagreements so that the group 'gets stuck' in a murky process.

4. Unclear contracts about time and sharing time, whose turn it is to present in supervision, case presentation formats and the general parameters of the group can lead to problems.

5. If one or more members is regularly absent, the life of the group will be affected.

6. The task may take predominance over time to reflect, to discuss and to play with new ideas.

7. The group may become too unstructured for effective learning to take place and may end up being a pleasant 'tea party'.

8. Finally, a group is a likely place for us to play out our familiar 'games' so it will be important to include in the contract a willingness to explore this process.

How to make the best of group supervision

The advantage of group supervision is that on many occasions there is an issue, a problem, or an area of work that all members wish to spend time reflecting upon. For example, we may agree that next time we will focus on 'the narcissistic process in individuals and in organisations' referring to examples from our own experience. This potential for shared learning is one of the best aspects of group supervision and maximises the benefit within the time constraints. Learning in a group may also serve to 'normalise' certain reactions that a person may be ashamed of or worried about owning. In general, members of supervision groups are at a similar level of experience and professional development so that all are assured that other members are likely to be struggling with some similar problems.

A group also provides us with an opportunity to share the work and experience of our peers in a confidential space that is not available elsewhere. This promotes an experience of 'twin-ship' that can be supportive to us as we learn and develop. In this way, being in a group supervision context provides an experience of a collaborative learning and a working environment that can provide a model for the workplace. It gives us the opportunity to interact with people whose learning styles and interpersonal styles may differ vastly from our own, and where such differences can be celebrated as a source of richness in life.

Simple steps to ensure you maximise your group experience

A group contract covering issues such as giving clear and honest feedback, an agreement not to hold on to 'bad feelings' but to air these in the group, and other aspects of emotional literacy is vital to the survival of a group. You are encouraged to raise this at the outset of the group so that all members are clear that this is an agreed norm.

If you have supervision in a group then people usually agree on an overall contract for the group which may involve agreements to give and receive honest feedback from all members of the group. All group members may also want a particular focus such as 'relating theoretical concepts to their practice' so this becomes an overall focus for the group. Then within the group, each person will contract session by session for what he/she wants from that session:

1.   **1st Person:** Today I want to review my relationship with a colleague and find a more creative way to work with her.

2.   **2nd Person:** I want to look at my work with a particular client and review my goals to see if they really fit the presenting problem.

3.   **3rd Person:** I have agreed to do a workshop and I would like to run through the design I have drawn up and get some input and feedback from the group.

These contracts are then worked on within the context of the group and keeping in mind the overall focus of the group. You can see from this that running a group is a balancing challenge for the supervisor!

A discussion of the time boundaries and how group members will be assured a fair share of the group time is essential. This agreement may differ from group to group in its details, but what you must ensure is that everyone feels satisfied that there is a balance in the group over the life of the group so that everyone gets their supervisory needs met satisfactorily.

Agreement as to the extent to which personal material is brought to the group, how this is done, and for what purpose is also an important discussion point that will need to be clarified for participants to feel comfortable and safe in a group.

Decide which aspects of your work you will be bringing to the group and make this clear from the outset. Make clear too what forms of presenting the material you will use and perhaps new ways you intend to experiment within the group. Remember, a group is a safe environment in which to experiment with new ways of presenting material, geared to enhancing your learning, e.g., through using audio recordings or asking to use role-plays.

Conclusion

The best book we know on Group Supervision is Proctor (2008). In it, she outlines four types of group supervision (authoritative, co-operative, participative and peer) and provides pathways and contracts within each to show how they compare and differ. This is an excellent reference.

Case example

How might the supervisor work with the following?

Your small supervision group is dealing with conflict. Two of the supervisees have formed an alliance and constantly defend each other and attack the third member of the group. You have tried to intervene to no avail. Now, they have started to attack you for not managing the group process.

Review and discussion

1. Can you articulate the advantages and disadvantages of group supervision?
2. What are the elements in group supervision that need to be considered if it is to be as effective as possible?
3. Could you draw up a group supervision contract? (See the contract in Appendix 1).

CHAPTER 16

Dealing with Problems in Supervision

While we hope your experience of supervision and of being a supervisee will be positive and contribute to your learning, we know there are times when problems in supervision make it a negative experience. Supervision is a co-operative endeavour and a relational learning process, and it is important that you feel comfortable with your supervisor and the process of the sessions. Furthermore, sometimes supervision is a triadic relationship between yourself, your supervisor *and* your organisation, whether that organisation is a training organisation or an employer.

Kaberry (1995), whose research on abuse in supervision mentioned earlier, shows how in some cases the supervisory alliance breaks down and is often irreparable. We wish to outline some possible problems and suggest precautionary measures to deal with conflict should it arise. Research in the USA, again with supervisees, reported that thirty-eight percent of those surveyed claimed there had been conflict in their supervision that interfered with their learning (Moskowitz & Rupert, 1983). There are two main conclusions worth noting from this research. The first finding was that there are three main areas of conflict: theoretical orientation, style of supervision and personality issues. Second, while the supervisees wanted their supervisors to monitor, identify and bring up the issues of disagreement, in fact eighty-three percent of supervisees had to initiate the discussion on the conflict. In this section, we will look at some of the most common areas where conflict arises (following the research findings listed above) and then consider some strategies that can be set in place for dealing with conflict should this arise.

Conflict related to theoretical orientation

Differences in theoretical orientation can lead to difficulties and conflict in supervision. In many agencies, supervisees may not have a choice of supervisor and may end up being supervised by someone who has a theoretical orientation different to their own. Usually such differences can be negotiated creatively and, as the supervisee, you can really benefit from a different perspective on the therapeutic process that may challenge some of your dearly-held assumptions. Since psychotherapy outcome research suggests consistently that there is no significant difference in outcome amongst different orientations (see Wampold, 2001), humility may be appropriate here! We can all learn from differences in perspective and enrich our own personal style by learning from others. Integration across orientations is also becoming more common, so nowadays it is easier to find a supervisor who comes from an integrative perspective and is used to talking across schools and orientations.

However, you may occasionally find that a supervisor is convinced of the 'rightness' of his/her orientation and is not prepared to accept interventions that arise from a different philosophy or school of psychology. He/she may even believe that what you are doing is harmful to the client although from your perspective it is well-aligned with your orientation. This difference will usually show up in relation to a particular style of intervention: for example, self-disclosure, which would be acceptable to gestaltists, existentialists and person-centred practitioners, might find less acceptance in the psychoanalytic tradition and be strongly contra-advised. This does not mean that any gratuitous self-disclosure is to be justified. Such a difference may be able to be 'held' within a supervisory alliance. Being open to hearing the supervisor's point of view about the possibly 'damaging' effects of a particular intervention or strategy could lead to rich learning and new ways of working.

However, it may also lead to conflict that cannot be resolved easily. Unfortunately, the history of counselling and psychotherapy has many examples of this kind of disagreement that led to rifts between people that were never healed. Occasionally this may happen to you as a supervisee. In such a case, it is probably best to find a context and a supervisor with whom you can negotiate differences of this kind. If people hold to their belief systems too dearly, negotiation may simply not be possible and withdrawal may be the better option.

Some approaches are more directive, others more non-directive and facilitative of dialogue. As different frameworks are linked with particular styles of intervention, it would be good for you to have a conversation about the assumptions that underpin the approach used by your supervisor. By doing so you will know what to expect and can assess as you progress whether this suits you. What is good to know is that there are different models of supervision and if one particular approach does not work for you, you can seek out a supervisor with a different orientation to the work. Interesting points to note: Do you prefer a supervisor who is active in asking questions, giving you homework and guiding the work as you go along with the use of checklists? Or do you respond better to a supervisor who listens and facilitates you to find your own solutions through reflection and exploration of your thoughts and feelings about the situation? Or someone who does both?

Good questions to ask are:

1. What kind of interventions (i.e., what does the supervisor do) are linked with this approach to the work?
2. What basic philosophy underpins the approach?
3. What would a typical supervision session look like?
4. What will be expected of each of us over the course of supervision?

These questions give you some idea of what to expect from the process of the sessions and from the supervision contract. You could then have an assessment period (e.g., three sessions) in which you can judge whether this approach is working for you and, at the review, make a decision about future sessions.

Conflict related to style of supervision

Supervisory styles differ just as personalities do! Some supervisors have a formal style while others are far more informal and relaxed in their approach. You may, for example, feel 'safer' with the person who is more formal, while a more relaxed style may leave you feeling too insecure. Or formality may inhibit you and you will learn better with a more informal approach. Rosenblatt and Meyer (cited in Albott, 1984) listed four unsatisfactory forms of supervision: *'constrictive supervision; amorphous supervision; unsupportive supervision; and 'therapeutic' supervision'* (p. 33).

In *'constrictive supervision'* there is limited autonomy, strictures on certain techniques, and innovation is frowned upon. In *'amorphous supervision'* there is little supervisory input and the supervisor may have a rather laissez-faire attitude to the whole process where 'anything goes'. In *'unsupportive supervision'* supervisors are aloof and distant and supervisees would not approach them readily with their difficulties. *'Therapeutic supervision'* turns the supervisee into a 'patient' while the supervisor takes on the role of the 'therapist' (with no contract to do so) often in an invasive and intrusive manner that infantilise the supervisee.

If we extrapolate from these findings, we can draw the following inferences: supervisees prefer supervisors (a) who allow exploration and experimentation, and are not rule-bound; (b) who balance facilitation of free discussion with supervisory input while holding boundaries around the task; (c) who are warm and supportive and therefore approachable; and (d) who do not use supervision as a vehicle for doing therapy with the supervisee but stick to the supervisory task and focus. Carifio and Hess (1987), following research into supervisory qualities came to this conclusion: *'The ideal supervisor is a person who shows respect, empathy, genuineness, concreteness and self-disclosure in his or her dealings with supervisees'* (p. 245).

The style of supervision can, of course, be negotiated and many supervisors will be open to discussing what you want more or less of in the sessions. Your needs may also change over time and then the style of the sessions can be renegotiated optimally to suit your stage of development and your current 'growing edges'.

Many of the people we have spoken to prefer a supervisor who balances support with confrontation in such a way that supervision does not become 'too cosy' or 'too belligerent'!

Conflict related to personality issues (relationship issues)

We sometimes hear of cases where there is a 'personality clash' between a supervisee and a supervisor which can lead to a break or rupture in the supervisory alliance. Such ruptures are often the result of misunderstandings in communication and you would be well-advised to raise such matters as soon as possible after they have arisen with a view to resolving the differences. It may happen that your supervisor misinterprets something you have said, or he/she may make a mistake about an appointment such as getting the time wrong or he/she may not have read something you sent in advance. Such mistakes are part of most relationships and are best resolved by open sharing of feelings and clearing up any misperceptions. It is important to share your disappointments, feelings and expectations so that your supervisor can understand what is important to you. Clear open communication is at the heart of effective supervision.

You also need to be alert to the occasions when the rupture may be due to your own defensiveness. For example, the supervisor may have given you feedback you experienced as hurtful or undermining, even though the supervisor may have tried to couch the feedback in as specific and helpful manner as possible. We all tend to be left with legacies from childhood in the form of beliefs about us that may be unhelpful (e.g., *"I am stupid; or inadequate; or selfish; or too demanding; or 'too much' for other people…"*). Something that the supervisor says may tap into our own negative belief system and we may go into a negative downward spiral without the supervisor even realising the unwitting impact of his/her statements. When you cannot sort this out by yourself, it may be best to bring the issue back to supervision and see if there is a 'grain of truth' in the criticism that has become all encompassing. What we are suggesting here is that both you and the supervisor can hold the responsibility for keeping the supervisory alliance open and well-functioning as a learning space for you.

Conflicts related to the contract(s)

There may be conflicts that arise because of a lack of clarity about the nature of the supervisory contract.

When a company hires a supervisor to work with supervisees and pays for the service, who is really the client? The supervisee? The company? Or both?

It is clear that the first loyalty of the supervisor is to the supervisee and to the clients with whom the supervisee works, but there is no simple answer to this problem if the company has hired the supervisor. Usually an organisation will expect that the supervision will relate to the work as it takes place in the context of the organisation (whether that organisation is a training one or one that employs the supervisee).

This becomes an issue if the aims of the supervision begin to diverge from the goals of the organisation. In a third-party contract of this kind, it is essential that clear contractual agreements are set in place at the start between the company representative, the supervisor and you as the supervisee. Such a contract would cover how any 'reporting' is done and what elements of the supervision would be up for discussion. However, not all problems can be foreseen and sometimes you may need to request a review of the contract if your needs no longer match those of the company. An associated problem is that of the boundaries of confidentiality. These need to be agreed clearly and set out at the start.

It is your right as a supervisee to know what, if any, information will be passed back to the company/organisation and exactly what information would fall into that category. A clear pre-emptive contract at the outset will mean that you know where you stand and how the three-cornered contract will operate. It is also important to establish how this information will be relayed; it is often best to set up an arrangement that involves joint meetings so that you are present at any discussions about yourself and your work. In this way, you will be part of any discussions related to the supervisory contract.

If you are worried or anxious about any part of the various coaching contracts agreed, then ask for clarification and, if needs be, for re-negotiation. It is important to get it right.

Evaluation problems

Carroll (1996), in discussing the tasks of supervision, points out that the evaluative task in supervision is the one where the power element is most clear: *'Evaluation does involve a power element. We cannot ignore that'*. The supervisor has to take seriously the task of evaluating the performance of the supervisee, making judgements about the effectiveness of the work in hand. Any critical or supportive feedback amounts to an evaluation. In general, supervisors distinguish between *formative* and *summative* evaluation. The formative evaluation involves the ongoing process of giving feedback; the summative evaluation, the report that needs to be written at the end of a year or for accreditation purposes. Problems can arise in either or both of these processes. For supervisors, it is a real challenge to balance the supportive and evaluative functions of their supervisory role and some do better than others at this process. You can make your contribution by making it possible for your supervisor regularly to give you both the 'good' and the 'bad' news by inviting comment on your work, e.g., *"What do you think that I could have done differently here"? "How would you judge my effectiveness in this session"?*

Problems in evaluation can take a variety of forms. A few examples follow:

1. You may disagree with feedback you receive on a piece of work and leave feeling 'misunderstood' and 'unappreciated' by your supervisor. (This calls for clarification and discussion when you next meet).

2. You may experience your supervisor as giving you sudden and unexpected negative feedback about an aspect of your work that seemed acceptable up to this point. (It may be that you have not been open to this feedback previously or that your supervisor now judges that you are ready for another challenge in terms of refining your work).

3. In the summative evaluation that may involve a supervisor's report for your course, your supervisor may find that your work is not yet of a standard for you to proceed with the training. This can be one of the most challenging times with a supervisor. You can learn a great deal from staying with your supervisor through this process and working with the points that he/she considers are your weaknesses. If you have had a good supervisory alliance in which you have received regular and balanced feedback, then this outcome should come as no surprise to you. However, if it does come as a surprise, then you may need to review how this has happened and discuss why you have not heard this news until the end of the year. Has there been some collusion between you and your supervisor to avoid negative feedback? Has your supervisor been 'hoping' that you will catch on eventually without expressing his/her doubts strongly enough?

Group problems

Supervision groups may throw up a variety of problems because of the very nature of the joint endeavour.

One of the main problems in group supervision is that it can turn into a process of 'individual supervision in the group' with the supervisor spending time with each person in turn without there being much interaction between members. This is simply not group supervision! If this happens it is best to raise this issue for discussion so that other members can give their points of view and the process can be eased up. Generally, the supervisor can act as a facilitator in this type of discussion.

Some group members may have known one another before the supervision group was set up and bring unresolved issues from their previous acquaintance into the group. These tensions may interfere with the alliance in the group and the process may become 'stuck' so that little constructive work can be done until these matters are brought out into the open, discussed and resolved. Clear contracts about future communication can prevent this process from recurring, e.g., an agreement to deal with any negative or 'paranoid' feelings as they arise.

Competitiveness between group members can create tensions in group supervision. This can involve competition around time and 'getting enough' which can be dealt with in different ways. Some groups carefully divide up the available time so that each member gets an equal share; others agree to a check-in period and then take turns. What is important here is that members get to understand the nature of the learning in group supervision. People learn from the presentations of others in addition to their own, so learning takes place *all the time* not just when you have your turn. There will also be issues that arise that are of interest or relevance to the whole group: it is a pity not to honour these as part of the group learning process and set time aside for these discussions.

Members may also compete for the attention and positive strokes from the supervisor and vie for attention in this way. Again this process is best brought out into the open and can raise the interesting issue of placing value on contributions from all of the group members which may not be honoured sufficiently in this competition. Members may also compete to be better than one another. Healthy competition where people stimulate one another to improve standards can be a productive feature of group supervision. However, it is counter-productive when members put one another down and undermine the other's work in order to aggrandise their own!

Vast differences in levels of competence can also create dissatisfaction in a group. It is generally better if members in a group are at more or less the same level of development, although it is possible with understanding and good facilitation for a group with varying levels of competence to function well as a learning community. In such cases the more experienced members could be of great help to the beginners and the beginners will all be bringing their own prior work and life experience into the group.

Critical moments in supervision

We do not want to end this section without dealing with the fact that all relationships hit crisis moments where ruptures and interruptions in the relationships raise their heads. These critical moments in the relationship are not necessarily signs that the relationship is heading for the rocks: at times they can be quite the opposite and are indicators that something needs review or that the relationship is being challenged to reach a new level and deal with a new factor. However, supervisees and supervisors sometimes panic when their relationship seems to hit an impasse or be blocked. Day, de Haan, Blass, Sills and Bertie (2008), in a fascinating piece of research, interviewed a number of executive coaches about critical moments in their coaching work and the use of supervision in helping them resolve these conflicts. We have adapted their work here to supervision. What they discovered was that critical moments in coaching are:

1. unforeseen;
2. bring heightened emotions;
3. give rise to tensions within the relationship.

These, in turn, give rise to anxiety and sometimes doubt on the part of the supervisor and the supervisee, which in turn result in potential opportunities for insight and change in the relationship or lead to a breakdown. It can be a 'make or break' situation. Day et al. (2008) isolated characteristics of these critical relationship moments:

1. heightened emotion for the supervisee;
2. heightened emotion for the supervisor, e.g., feelings of anger, fear, sadness, doubts, inadequacy;
3. a tension or tension in the relationship (a crossroads).

They outline steps/stages in the process involved in the emergence of critical moments in coaching:

1. All moments start with action or raw emotion.
2. Counteractions—often a defensive reaction: an immediate, unprocessed response.
3. Interior dialogue (or internal ethical dilemma). This is thinking-after-the-event. A distancing.
4. Explicit distancing in the relationship (not turning up).
5. Shared reflection—explore the state of their own relationship.
6. Deepening of the relationship (sometimes re-contracting).
7. Satisfactory change for the supervisee (often new insights).
8. Breakdown of the relationship.
9. Unknown future.

What the researchers found made the difference between whether or not the relationship continues depends on the kind of interventions used by the supervisor. These included:

1. Confronting or challenging the supervisee with interest and acceptance.
2. Providing feedback to the supervisee in the 'here-and-now' about what was happening.
3. Sharing their own feelings with the supervisee.
4. Reflecting on the possible link to the supervisee's issues and feelings.
5. Helping the supervisee to clarify their thinking.
6. Providing direction.

Supervisors and supervisees need not back away from these moments of rupture—they can choose to stay with them and make them into 'generative moments' in their supervisory relationship. We mention their research to encourage you to stay with awkward, difficult or challenging moments in supervision in order to see if these moments are asking both you and your supervisor to deepen the relationship and face new challenges. On the other hand, we want you to be alert to the signs that your supervisory relationship might be at an end, or that it would be unhelpful for you to continue it. Knowing the difference is quite a skill and often comes with experience and practice.

Setting in place strategies for dealing with conflict

When setting up a supervisory contract, it is worthwhile to set in place strategies for dealing with any potential conflict. These may include the following steps, some preventative, and some palliative:

1. Sometimes it is good to start by approaching conflicts as opportunities for learning and not necessarily as breakdowns in relationships. When we ask: *"What is this conflict really about and what role am I playing in it?"*, we can often find conflict a great source of learning.

2. At the outset, express your expectations of supervision very clearly and request the same of the supervisor so that you are both clear about what is expected on both sides.

3. Make a contract that focuses on your learning goals for the duration of the initial contract (usually these are made year by year) and also come to each supervision session with a clear focus on what you wish to gain from the session.

4. Suggest a mutual agreement to give regular ongoing feedback to one another about the process of supervision.

5. Agree to regular reviews every few weeks to refer back to the overall goals of supervision.

6. Make an agreement with yourself to raise any area of conflict when it arises (or as soon as possible after the event) and not to let it fester and get worse over time!

7. If there is conflict, first try to sort this out directly with your supervisor. It is a good idea to set aside a certain amount of time on a regular basis to talk about issues of conflict. You would also be well-advised to set out in advance the points you wish to discuss so that you are both clear about the agenda for the meeting. That way you will be able to focus on the central conflict area/s.

8. If it proves impossible for you and your supervisor to resolve the matter or the rupture seems to be widening, suggest that you approach a third person to act as mediator. This would generally be someone from outside your systems, but a person you both feel you could work with. At best, this process could lead to a resolution and clarity about how you move forward; or, at worst, it may facilitate a parting between the two of you without rancour and resentment. Since we are part of common professional bodies and may well meet up at conferences, etc., it is important to reach a stage when you can meet in public without discomfort.

It is good to realise that sometimes certain relationships do not work and that is that.

Your supervisor will probably belong to a professional organisation, subscribe to a code of ethics and have indemnity insurance for his or her supervision work. If you felt your supervisor was or has been unethical or seriously unprofessional, then it is possible to make a complaint or take out an ethical charge against him or her. Such an action would not be taken lightly but it does remain another possible way of dealing with conflict areas in supervision. Your supervisor will be able to provide you with a copy of the Code of Ethics (or the Ethical Framework) to which he/she subscribes and the Professional Body of which he/she is a member.

Conclusion

While we have looked at some conflicts that may arise within supervision we have, by no means, listed all possible difficulties. It is worthwhile being prepared for when relationships go wrong, for whatever reason. Overall, we hope that through talking about the differences that they can become sources of learning. If need be, having others involved to help us resolve difficulties is simply an acknowledgement that there are times when we need referees and observers who have an 'outside' stance regarding our 'inside' way of seeing what is taking place.

Review and discussion

1. What do you think is the best way to deal with conflicts in relationships? Can you think of an example from your own personal or professional environment where you have had to resolve a difference or difficulty? What would you do differently now?

2. What makes conflict in relationships (and in particular in the supervisory relationship), and dealing with conflict, a difficult process?

Conclusion to the Manual

You have come to the end of the formal part of this manual. Our hope is that you have worked out for yourself a philosophy of supervision (what it means), that you have a clear format for negotiating a contract within supervision, and that you have methodologies and frameworks for preparing for and presenting within supervision. We hope, too, that you have built in antennae that will alert you to potential difficulties within supervision and also keep you aware of the processes underlying all aspects of supervision. With those in place, we feel sure that your supervision will be a dynamic place of learning and the end result with be a qualitatively different service for your client group.

References and Further Reading

Albott, W. L. (1984). Supervisory characteristics and other sources of supervision variance. In T. H. Peake & R. P. Archer (Eds.), *Clinical Training in Psychotherapy* (pp. 27–43). Binghamton, NY: The Haworth Press.

Bateson, G. (2000). *Steps to ecology of mind: Collected essays in anthropology, psychiatry, evolution, and epistemology.* Chicago: University of Chicago Press.

Bambling, M. (2009). Alliance supervision to enhance client outcomes. In N. Pelling, J. Barletta, & P. Armstrong (Eds.), *The Practice of Clinical Supervision* (pp. 121–137). Bowen Hills, Queensland: Australian Academic Press.

Belenky, M., Clinchy, B., Goldberger, N., & Tarule, J. (1986). *Women's ways of knowing: The development of self, voice, and mind.* New York: Basic Books.

Berger, S. & Buchholz, E. (1993). On being a supervisee: Preparation for learning in a supervisory relationship. *Psychotherapy: Theory, Research, Practice, Training, 30*(1), 86–92.

Bolton, G. (2001). *Reflective practice: Writing and professional development.* London: Paul Chapman.

Bond, M. & Holland, S. (1998). *Skills of clinical supervision for nurses.* Buckingham: Open University Press.

Boud, D., Keogh, R., & Walker, D. (Eds.). (1985). *Reflection: Turning experience into learning.* London: Kogan Page.

Brockbank, A. & McGill, I. (1998). *Facilitating reflective learning in higher education.* Buckingham: Open University Press.

Brew, A. (1993). Unlearning through experience. In D. Boud, R. Cohen, & D. Walker (Eds.), *Using experience for learning* (pp. 87–98). Buckingham: Open University Press.

Campbell, J. M. (2000). *Becoming an effective supervisor: A workbook for counselors and psychotherapists.* Philadelphia: Taylor & Francis Group.

Carifio, M. & Hess, A. (1987). Who is the ideal supervisor? *Professional Psychology: Research and Practice, 18*(3), 244–250.

Carroll, M. (2004). *Awake at work: 35 practical Buddhist principles for discovering clarity and balance in the midst of work's chaos.* Boston: Shambhala Press.

Carroll, M. (2009). From mindless to mindful practice: Learning reflection in supervision. *Psychotherapy in Australia, 15*(4), 38–49.

Carroll, M. (2007). Coaching supervision: Luxury or necessity? In S. Palmer, & A. Whybrow (Eds.), *The handbook of coaching psychology: A guide for practitioners.* London: Routledge.

Carroll, M. (2005). Psychological contracts with and within organisations. In R. Tribe & M. Morrissey (Eds.), *Professional and ethical issues for psychologists, psychotherapists and counsellors* (pp. 33–47). London: Brunner-Routledge.

Carroll, M. (1996). *Counselling supervision: Theory, skills and practice.* London: Cassell.

Carroll, M., & Holloway, E. (Eds.). (1999). *Counselling supervision in context.* London: Sage Publications.

Carroll, M., & Tholstrup, M. (Eds.). (2001). *Integrative approaches to supervision.* London: Jessica Kingsley.

Casement, P. (1985). *On learning from the patient.* London: Tavistock.

Clarkson, P., & Gilbert, M. (1991). The training of counsellor trainers and supervisors. In W. Dryden & B. Thorne (Eds.), *Training and supervision for counselling in action.* London: Sage Publications.

Claxton, G. (1999). *Wise up: The challenge of lifelong learning.* New York, NY: Bloomsbury Publishing.

Connor, M., & Pokora, J. (2007). *Coaching and mentoring at work: Developing effective practice.* Maidenhead, Berkshire: Open University Press.

Coupland, D. (1991). *Generation X: Tales for an accelerated culture.* London: Abacus.

Copeland, S. (2005). *Counselling supervision in organisations: Professional and ethical dilemmas explored.* London: Routledge.

Day, A., de Haan, E., Blass, E., Sills, C. & Bertie, C. (2008). Critical moments in the coaching relationship: Does supervision help? *International Coaching Psychology Review, 3*(3), 207–218.

Derrida. J. (1981). *Positions.* Chicago: The University of Chicago Press.

Dewey, J. (1933). *How we think: A restatement of the relation of reflective thinking to the educative process* (Rev. ed.). Boston: D. C. Heath.

Dixon, N. (1998). *Dialogue at work.* London: Lemos and Crane.

Ellis, M. (2010). Bridging the science and practice of clinical supervision: Some discoveries, some misconceptions. *The Clinical Supervisor, 29*(1), 95–116.

Enright, R. (2001). *Forgiveness is a choice: A step-by-step process for resolving anger and restoring hope.* Washington, DC. American Psychological Association.

Fine, C. (2007). *A mind of its own.* London: Icon Books.

Freire, P. (1998). *Teachers as cultural workers.* Oxford: Westview Press.

Gardner, H. (1999). *Intelligence reframed: Multiple intelligences for the 21st century.* New York, NY: Basic Books.

Gelb, M. (1999). *How to think like Leonardo da Vinci: Seven steps to genius everyday.* New York, NY: Dell Publishing.

Gilbert, D. (2006). *Stumbling on happiness.* London: Harper Press.

Gilbert, M. & Evans, K. (2000). *Psychotherapy supervision: An integrative relational approach to psychotherapy supervision.* Buckingham: Open University Press.

Gilbert, M. & Sills, C. (1999). Training for supervision evaluation. In E. Holloway & M. Carroll (Eds.), *Training counselling supervisors: Strategies, methods and techniques* (pp. 162–84). London: Sage Publications.

Goleman, D. (1996). *Emotional intelligence: Why it can matter more than IQ.* London: Blooomsbury Publishing.

Goleman, D. (1998). *Working with Emotional Intelligence.* London: Bloomsbury Publishing.

Hawkins, P., & Smith, N. (2006). *Coaching, mentoring and organisational consultancy: Supervision and development.* Maidenhead, UK: Open University Press.

Hawkins, P. & Shohet, R. (1989). *Supervision in the helping professions.* Milton Keynes: Open University Press.

Hawkins, P. & Shohet, R. (2000). *Supervision in the helping professions* (2nd ed.). Milton Keynes: Open University Press.

Hawkins, P. & Shohet, R. (2007). *Supervision in the helping professions* (3rd ed.). Milton Keynes: Open University Press.

Hazell, J. W. (1989). Drivers as mediators of stress response. *Transactional Analysis Journal, 19*(4), 212–223.

Henderson, P. (2009). *A different wisdom: Reflections on supervision practice*. London: Karnac Books.

Hewson, J. (1999). Training supervisors to contract in supervision. In E. Holloway & M. Carroll (Eds.), *Training counselling supervisors: Strategies, methods and techniques* (pp. 67¬–92). London: Sage Publications.

Holloway, E. (1995). *Clinical supervision: A systems approach*. Thousand Oaks, CA: Sage Publications.

Holloway, E. & Carroll, M. (Eds.). (1999). *Training counselling supervisors: Strategies, methods and techniques*. London: Sage Publications.

Holton, G. & Benefiel, M. (Eds.). (2010). *The soul of supervision: Integrating practice and theory*. New York, NY: Morehouse Publishing.

Honey, P. & Mumford, A. (1992). *The manual of learning styles*. Maidenhead: Peter Honey Publications.

Horton, I. (1993). Supervision. In R. Bayne & P. Nicolson (Eds.), *Counselling and psychology for health professionals* (pp. 28–31). London: Chapman and Hall.

Horton, M., Kohl, J., & Kohl, H. (1990). *The long haul: An autobiography*. New York, NY: Doubleday Books.

Huston, T. (2007). *Inside out: Stories and methods for generating collective will to create the future we want*. Cambridge, MA: The Society for Organisational Learning.

Houston, G. (1990). *Supervision and counselling*. London: Rochester Foundation.

Inskipp, F. (1999). Training supervisees to use supervision. In E. Holloway & M. Carroll (Eds.), *Training counselling supervisors: Strategies, methods and techniques* (pp. 184–211). London: Sage Publications.

Inskipp, F. & Proctor, B. (1993). *Art, craft and tasks of counselling supervision. Professional development for counsellors, psychotherapists, supervisors and trainees, Pt. 1: Making the most of supervision*. Middlesex, UK: Cascade Publications.

Inskipp, F. & Proctor, B. (1995). *Art, craft and tasks of counselling supervision. Professional development for counsellors, psychotherapists, supervisors and trainees, Pt. 2: Becoming a supervisor*. Middlesex, UK: Cascade Publications.

Inskipp, F. & Proctor, B. (2001). *Art, craft and tasks of counselling supervision. Professional development for counsellors, psychotherapists, supervisors and trainees, Pt. 2: Becoming a supervisor* (2nd ed.). Middlesex, UK: Cascade Publications.

Isaacs, W. (1999). *Dialogue and the art of thinking together: A pioneering approach to communicating in business and in life.* New York, NY. Doubleday Books.

Jarvis, P. (2006). *Towards a comprehensive theory of human learning.* London: Routledge.

Kaberry, S. (1995). *Abuse in supervision.* (M. Ed. Dissertation, University of Birmingham, UK).

Kahler, T., & Capers, H. (1974). The miniscript. *Transactional Analysis Journal,* 4(1), 26–42.

Kahler, T. (1978). *Transactional analysis revisited.* Little Rock: Human Development Publications.

Kaufman, G. (1992). *Shame: The power of caring* (3rd ed.). Rochester, VT: Schenkman Books.

Kagan, N. (1980). Influencing human interaction: Eighteen years with IPR. In A. K. Hess (Ed.), *Psychotherapy supervision: Theory, research and practice* (pp. 262–286). New York: Wiley.

Kegan, R. (1994). *In over our heads: The mental demands of modern life.* Cambridge, MA: Harvard University Press.

Kegan, R., & Lahey, L. L. (2009). *Immunity to change: How to overcome it and unlock the potential in yourself and your organization.* Boston: Harvard Business Press.

King, P. M., & Kitchener. L. S. (1994). *Developing reflective judgement.* San Francisco, CA: Jossey-Bass.

Kline, N. (1999). *Time to think: Listening to ignite the human mind.* London: Ward Lock & Co.

Knapman, J., & Morrison, T. (1998). *Making the most of supervision in health and social care: A self-development manual for supervisees.* Brighton, UK: Pavilion Publishing.

Knibb, J. (2010). *Special children: Mothering matters* (Doctoral Dissertation, University of Bristol, Graduate School of Education, UK).

Kolb, D. (1984). *Experiential learning: Experience as the source of learning and development.* Englewood Cliffs, NJ: Prentice Hall.

Lahad, M. (2000). *Creative supervision: The use of expressive arts methods in supervision and self-supervision.* London: Jessica Kingsley Publishers.

Lammers, W. (1999). Training in group and team supervision. In E. Holloway & M. Carroll (Eds.), *Training counselling supervisors: Strategies, methods and techniques* (pp. 106–130). London: Sage Publications.

Langer, E. (1989). *Mindfulness.* Cambridge, MA: Cambridge University Press.

Law, H., Ireland, S., & Hussain, Z. (2007). *The psychology of coaching, mentoring and learning.* Chichester, UK: John Wiley & Sons.

Leary, M. R. (2004). *The curse of the self: Self-awareness, egotism, and the quality of human life.* New York, NY: Oxford University Press.

Marsick, V. J., & Maltbia, T. E. (2009). The transformative potential of action learning conversations: Developing critically reflective practice skills. In J. Mezirow, E. Taylor, & Associates (Eds.), *Transformative learning in practice: Insights from community, workplace and higher education.* San Francisco, CA: Jossey-Bass.

May, S. E., & O'Donovan, A. (2007). The advantages of the mindful therapist. *Psychotherapy in Australia, 13*(4), 46–53.

McAlpine, L., & Weston, C. (2002). Reflection, improving teaching and students learning. In N. Hativa & P. Goodyear (Eds.), *Teacher thinking, beliefs and knowledge in higher education.* Dordrecht, Netherlands: Kluwer Academic Publishers.

McLaughlin, J. T. (2005). *The healer's bent: Solitude and dialogue in the clinical encounter.* Hillsdale, NJ: The Analytic Press.

Mezirow, J., & Associates (2000). *Learning as transformation: Critical perspectives on a theory in progress.* San Francisco, CA: Jossey-Bass.

Mezirow, J., Taylor, E., & Associates (Eds.). (2009). *Transformative learning in practice: Insights from community, workplace and higher education.* San Francisco, CA: Jossey-Bass.

Milne, D. (2009). *Evidence-based clinical supervision: Principles and practice.* Chichester, West Sussex: BPS Blackwell.

Moloney, K. (2005). The frog prince: Giving tips on how to choose a coach. *Coaching at Work, 1*(1), 51–55.

Moon, J. (1999). *Reflection in learning and professional development: Theory and practice.* London: Kogan Page.

Moon, J. (2004). *A handbook of reflective and experiential learning: Theory and practice.* London: Routledge Falmer.

Moore, B. (2008). *Group supervision with a multi-disciplinary trauma resource team in the north of Ireland: A participative inquiry into the application of a 'process framework'.* D. Prof. Middlesex University, London.

Moskowitz, S. A., & Rupert, P. A. (1983). Conflict resolution within the supervisory relationship. *Professional Psychology: Research and Practice, 14,* 632–641.

Murphy, K. (2009). *Keynote address at the British Association for Supervision Practice and Research.* London, July.

Neufeldt. S. (1999). Training in reflective processes in supervision. In E. Holloway & M. Carroll (Eds.), *Training counselling supervisors: Strategies, methods and techniques* (pp. 92–106). London: Sage Publications.

Ofman, D. (2001). *Core qualities: A gateway to human resources.* Netherlands: Scriptum Publishers.

Orme, G. (2001). *Emotionally intelligent living.* Glasgow: Crown House Publishing.

Ostell, A., Baverstock, S., & Wright, P. (1999). Interpersonal skills of managing emotion at work. *The Psychologist, 12*(1), 30–35.

Pampallis-Paisley, P. (2006). *Towards a theory of supervision for coaching: An integral approach.* D. Prof. Middlesex University, London.

Proctor, B. (2008). *Group supervision: A guide to creative practice* (2nd ed.). London: Sage Publications.

Queneau, R. (1947/1998). *Exercises in style.* London: John Calder Publishing.

Ray, M., & Myers, R. (1986). *Creativity in business.* New York, NY: Broadway Books.

Robinson, W. L. (1974). Conscious competency: The mark of the competent instructor. *Personnel Journal, 53,* 538–539.

Rock, D. (2006). *Quiet leadership: Six steps to transforming performance at work.* New York: Harper Collins.

Rogers, C. (2004). *On becoming a person: A therapist's view of psychotherapy.* London: Constable.

Rokeach, M. (1979). *Understanding human values.* New York: Simon and Schuster .

Ryan, S. (2004). *Vital practice: Stories from the healing arts. The homeopathic and supervisory way.* Portland, UK: Sea Change Publications.

Sartre, J. P. (2003). *Being and nothingness: An essay on phenomenological ontology.* London: Routledge.

Scharmer, C. O. (2007). *Theory U: Leading from the future as it emerges.* Cambridge, MA: Society for Organizational Learning.

Schon, D. (1983). *The reflective practitioner: How professionals think in action.* New York: Basic Books.

Schon, D. (1987). *Educating the reflective practitioner.* San Francisco, CA: Jossey-Bass.

Siegel, D. J. (2007). *The mindful brain: Reflection and attunement in the cultivation of well-being.* New York, NY: W. W. Norton.

Smith, A. (1998). *Accelerated learning in practice.* Stafford: Network Educational Press.

Stoltenberg, C. D., & McNeill, B. W. (2010). *IDM Supervision: An integrated development model for supervising counselors and therapists.* New York, NY: Routledge.

Strenger, C. (2005). *The designed self: Psychoanalysis and contemporary identities.* London: The Analytic Press.

Tannenbaum, S. (1997). Enhancing continuous learning: Diagnostic findings from multiple companies. *Human Resource Management, 36*(4), 437–452.

Vaill, P. (1996). *Learning as a way of being: Strategies for survival in a world of permanent white water.* San Francisco: Jossey-Bass.

Vespia, K. M., Hechman-Stone, C. & Delwith, U. (2002). Describing and facilitating effective supervison behaviour in counselling trainees. *Psychotherapy: Theory, Research, Practice, Training, 39*(1), 56–65.

Voller, H. (2010). *Developing the understanding of reflective practice in counselling and psychotherapy.* D. Prof, University of Middlesex.

Wampold, B. (2001). *The great psychotherapy debate: Models, methods, and findings.* New Jersey: Lawrence Erlbaum Associates.

Weisinger, H. (1998). *Emotional intelligence at work.* San Francisco: Jossey-Bass.

Zachary, L. (2002). *The mentor's guide: Facilitating effective learning relationships.* San Francisco: Jossey-Bass.

Zohar, D., & Marshall, I. (2001). *Spiritual intelligence: The ultimate intelligence.* London: Bloomsbury Publishing.

Zuboff, S., & Maxmin, J. (2002). *The support economy: Why corporations are failing individuals and the next episode of capitalism.* New York, NY: Viking Penguin.

Appendix 1: Example of a Two-way Supervision Contract

(Please note that this contract is taken from a counselling supervision arrangement and would need to be adapted to other professional contexts.)

This is a supervision contract:

Between _____ and _____

from _____ until its review (or ending) on _____

We both:

1.   are members of BACP (British Association for Counselling and Psychotherapy).
2.   abide by their Code of Ethics and Practice.
3.   have indemnity insurance for our work.

What is supervision?

We are agreed that supervision is a forum used by supervisees to reflect on all aspects of their clinical work, where they receive formal and informal feedback on that work and where the welfare of clients and the quality of the service they receive is central.

Practicalities:

We will meet for _____ hours every _____ at a time to be arranged at the end of each supervisory session. Ours is a non-smoking environment and we have agreed that each of us will ensure that there are no unnecessary interruptions (mobiles, phone, people).

(Add here anything about groups if group supervision, or fees, if necessary, or equipment, e.g., flip charts, overhead projects, video, audio, etc.).

Procedures:

We have agreed that the following arrangements will take place in the following situations:

Cancellation of session

Non-attendance at supervision session

Where there are disagreements, disputes, conflict areas between supervisor/supervisee(s)

If there is need for extra supervision

Contracts with others, e.g., an organisation or a training course

---

For appeals

Keeping of supervisory notes

Emergencies (you are free to phone me if there is an emergency on the following number _____).

What will you (supervisee) do if I (the supervisor) am not available?

Guidelines:

The following guidelines/ground rules will guide our time together:

1. Confidentiality (what we mean by confidentiality is)…

    ---

2. Openness/honesty (about work done, the supervisory relationship, reports, etc.).
3. Line management issues that may pertain (especially if the supervisor is also the line-manager).
4. Gossip (any leakage of information in the systems).
5. Using feedback to learn.

Roles and responsibilities:

We have agreed that as supervisor I will take responsibility for:

1. Time keeping.

2. Managing the overall agenda of sessions.
3. Giving feedback.
4. Monitoring the supervisory relationship.
5. Creating a safe place.
6. Monitoring ethical issues of counselling and supervision.
7. Keeping notes of sessions.
8. Drawing up the final supervisory reports.

We have agreed that as supervisee you will be responsible for:

1. Preparing for supervision.
2. Presenting in supervision.
3. Your learning (objectives); applying learning from supervision.
4. Feedback to self and to supervisor.
5. Keeping notes of supervisory sessions.

Evaluation and Review:

We have agreed that informal evaluation of:

1. supervisee;
2. supervisor;
3. supervision.

will take place every sixth session. Formal Evaluations will take place every year or as requested by either supervisor or supervisee.

The criteria against which evaluation of supervisees will take place are at the end of this contract.

Formal reports will be sent to _____

and can be viewed by _____

They will be kept at _____

The process for formal evaluation of supervisees (written) will be:

1. Self evaluation by supervisee.
2. Evaluation by supervisor.
3. Initial report by supervisor to be seen and commented on by supervisee.
4. Final report written by supervisor with space for comments by supervisee.
5. Report sent to agreed personnel (above).

Re-negotiation of Contract:

At any time either party (supervisor and/or supervisee) can initiate discussion around re-negotiation of the contract or any part of it. This will be done in advance so there is preparatory time available.

Signed: _____ (Supervisor)

Signed: _____ (Supervisee/s)

Signed: _____ (Others, e.g., organisation or training institute)

Criteria for evaluating the supervisee

The helping relationship:

1. Is the supervisee able to establish an effective relationship?
2. Does the supervisee engage with clients?
3. Does the supervisee use power appropriately?

Awareness of self:

1. Is the supervisee aware of themselves and their own strengths/limits?
2. Is the supervisee reflective?

Skills/competencies:

1. Does the supervisee have the skills of self-presentation?
2. Of listening/responding/of effective challenge?

Understanding the helping process:

1. Does the supervisee understand what is happening between self and client?
2. Is the supervisee aware of the stages of helping?

Diagnosis/assessment:

1. Has the supervisee a method of assessing/diagnosing clients?
2. Is the supervisee able to make clear and accurate diagnosis?

Contextual issues:

1. Is the supervisee aware of contextual issues in helping?
2. Is the supervisee aware of individual differences?

Ethics/professionalism:

1. Does the supervisee have a clear code of ethics to which they subscribe?
2. Is the supervisee ethically sensitive to what happens in helping?

Theory:

1. Does the supervisee have a theory that guides their work?
2. Is the supervisee congruent in theory and practice?
3. Has the supervisee sufficient knowledge to back up practice?

Attitudes, beliefs, values:

1. Is the supervisee flexible?

2. Is the supervisee tolerant and able to stay with painful issues?
3. Is the supervisee able to learn from supervision?
4. Does the supervisee deal positively with feedback?

Appendix 2: Supervision Session Evaluation Form

What in particular went well in our supervision session?

_____

What relationship challenges did we face?

_____

Were we communicating effectively with each other?

_____

Were we candid and open in our communication?

_____

What did we not talk about (avoided)?

_____

What learning challenges emerged?

_____

Any external factors that impacted on our supervision session?

_____

What three actions could improve the quality of our supervision arrangement:

a)

_____

b)

_____

c)

_____

Date _____

Appendix 3: An Evaluation Feedback Form for Supervisees

Am I (your supervisor) providing sufficient support to facilitate your learning?

_____

Have we identified sufficient and varied opportunities for your learning?

_____

Is the supervision relationship productive? Is there anything we need to discuss?

_____

Is the feedback I give thoughtful, candid and constructive?

_____

Is there a good balance of support and challenge in our supervision?

_____

Are there areas we do not talk about that should be the focus of a conversation?

_____

Is what we are discussing in supervision having an impact on your performance in life or work?

_____

What seems to you to be the next challenge in your development?

_____

What is most helpful about our supervision arrangement? What is least helpful?

_____

Is there anything you would like me to stop doing, start doing, increase or decrease?

_____

Are we being accountable in our supervision? To clients? To relevant organisation? To our profession?

_____

Date _____

Appendix 4: A Model for Ethical Decision Making for Supervisees

Stage 1: Creating ethical sensitivity (watchfulness)

Stage 1 is a good way to create ethical sensitivity so that you are aware (mindful and watchful) of what might be a professional or ethical issue. The following suggestions are ways to heighten your awareness of when you may need to consider an action or event as ethical:

1. Case reviews (go back over some of the dilemmas you have faced in your work).
2. Identify ethical issues arising from your work.
3. Read ethical codes and related literature.
4. Case vignettes (*"What would you do if...?"* and here create some difficult situations).
5. Exploring value-issues arising from work.
6. Clarifying and confronting one's own values.
7. Creating awareness around the 'power' issues involved in your work.
8. Reviewing critical incidents you, or others, have experienced.
9. Evaluating ethical frameworks and theories.
10. Ascertaining levels of moral development and how this affects ethical decision-making.

Stage 2: Formulating an ethical course of action

Stage 2 (with its seven steps) will help you formulate an ethical course of action where you are faced with what looks like needing an ethical decision.

Identify the ethical problem, or dilemma

1. What are the parameters of the situation?
2. What is the source of conflict for yourself and others involved?
3. Is the conflict with another person, group of people, or family member, or with the organisation?
4. Is the conflict between you and another person?
5. Does the conflict involve legal, moral, ethical, religious, cultural, gender, or value issues?
6. What are your feelings about what is happening?

7. How may the problem be defined clearly, especially where terms are emotionally charged?

Identify the potential issues involved

1. What is the worst possible outcome?
2. What could happen if nothing is done?
3. What are the implications involved in this problem or dilemma?
4. What are the rights, responsibilities, and welfare of all affected parties?

Review the relevant ethical guidelines

5. Do guidelines, principles, or laws exist that are relevant to the dilemmas and may provide a possible solution?
6. Are your values, ethics, or morals in conflict with the relevant principles or guidelines?
7. Are you aware of the effect of values and do you have a rationale for the behaviour?
8. Are there relevant codes, sections, chapters of books, etc., pertinent to this issue?
9. What further information is needed to help resolve the issues?

Obtain consultation

1. Bring the situation to supervision.
2. Talk with colleagues, where appropriate.
3. Consult line-managers, if appropriate.
4. Talk to a lawyer (or an expert from another profession), again if appropriate.

Consider possible and probable courses of action

1. What are the alternatives? (brainstorming without evaluating is helpful).

Enumerate the consequences of various decisions

1. What are the implications for the client?
2. What are the implications for others?
3. What are the implications for you?

Decide on what appears to be the best course of action

1. Could you recommend this action to others in similar circumstances?
2. Would I condone what you are about to do in another supervisee?

3. Can you defend this behaviour if it were made public?
4. Would I treat others in the same situation differently, i.e., from the decision I have made about this person or these people?

Stage 3: Implementing an ethical decision

Stage 3 is about taking steps to implement what you have decided. It is noteworthy that many people know what to do ethically and still do not implement their decision.

1. What steps need to be taken to implement the decision?
2. What people are involved and who needs to be told what?
3. What restraints are there to not implement the ethical decision (e.g., politics of the situation, protection of a client, rationalisation, etc.)?
4. What support is needed (by you, by others) to implement and to live with the results?

Stage 4: Living with the ambiguities of having made the decision

Making ethical decisions does not always mean you are happy with the results. Sometimes you have to live with the dilemma of not ever knowing if your decision was the best. However, you have made it in the light of the best information and consultation available to you. You will still have to consider:

1. Dealing with anxiety around the final decision.
2. Letting go of the situation and the dilemma.
3. Accepting the limitations involved.
4. Formulating learning from the experience.
5. Using personal and professional support to live with the consequences of the decision.

Appendix 5: A Supervisory Note Taking Format

Supervision Session Report

Supervisor: _____

Supervisee: _____

Date: _____

Issues raised in supervision:

_____

_____

Client Issues:

_____

Intervention issues:

_____

Supervisee Issues:

_____

Supervisor issues:

_____

Organisational Issues:

_____

Training Issues:

_____

Action points:

_____

_____

Signed: _____

Appendix 6: A Case Example Presentation in Supervision

Identification

1. A first name only, gender, age group, life stage.
2. Your first impressions. Physical appearance.

Antecedents

1. How the client came to see you, e.g., self-referral.
2. Context/location, e.g., agency, private practice, hospital, clinic.
3. Pre-contact information. What you knew about the client before you first met. How you used this information. Any existing relationship or previous contact with the client and possible implications.

Presenting problem and contact

1. Summary of the client's presenting problem.
2. Your initial assessment. Duration of problem. Precipitating factors (i.e., why the client came at this point). Current conflicts or issues.
3. Contract. Frequency, length and number of sessions. Initial plan.

Questions for supervision

1. Key question(s) or issues you want to discuss in supervision.

Focus on content

1. Client's account of problem situation:
   A. Work—significant activity, interests. How client spends his/her time and energy.
   B. Relationships—significant people, family and friends.
   C. Identity—self-concept, feelings and attitudes about self.
   D. Additional related or explanatory elements might include client's past/ early experiences; strengths and resources; beliefs and values; hopes, fears and fantasies. Possible implications of cultural, economic, social, political and other systems.
2. Problem definition:
   A. Construct a picture of the client's view of the present scenario.
   B. What is the client's preferred scenario? What would the client like to happen? How would the client like things to be?
3. Assessment and reformulation—how you account for and explain the presenting problem:

A. Patterns/strands/themes/connections that emerge.

B. In what way are these things important to explore?

C. What theoretical concepts/models or explanatory frameworks can be used for assessment? What hunches, new perspectives?

D. What else has not been mentioned that might be important to explore? What silent hypotheses, blind spots? What underlying issues or past problems?

4. Counselling plan:

   A. What direction or focus for future work? What possibilities, agenda?

   B. What criteria for change: theoretical frameworks and assumptions?

   C. View and/or reformulate plan(s).

Focus on process

1. Strategies and Interventions:

   A. What strategies and interventions have you used?

   B. What were you trying to achieve?

   C. What was the effect on the client?

   D. Generate alternative options.

2. Relationship:

   A. What happened between you and the client?

   B. Describe the relationship: reframe relationship; try a metaphor.

   C. What was happening within the client (transference)?

   D. What was happening within you (countertransference)?

   E. What changes have there been within the developing relationship over the period being discussed?

   F. Evaluate the 'working alliance'.

3. Evaluation:

   A. Review process.

   B. Consider alternative tasks, strategies and ways to implement counselling plan.

Focus on parallel process

1. What was happening between you and the supervisor?

2. Any parallels? What thoughts, feelings, experiences? Does what was going on in the supervisory relationship tell you anything about what may have been going on between you and the client?

Critical incident analysis

1. Description:
    A. What did the client say or do at that particular point?
    B. What did you say or do?
    C. How did the client respond to your interventions?
    D. What was happening within you?

2. Analysis:
    A. What was happening within the client?
    B. What was going on between you and the client?
    C. Intention and impact of interventions/responses.
    D. What hunches/hypotheses did you/do you have?
    E. Review. Any further/alternative perspectives, strategies and interventions.

Listening to aspects of covert communication

1. What was happening within you? How well can you listen to your own emotional response to a client? You may be aware of your feelings first and your thoughts later. Reflection on your emotional experience may help you gain information about what part of the client is likely to be in need of change. A simple way to use yourself as a measuring instrument is to ask:
    A. How does this client make me feel?
    B. What does the client say and do so that I feel the way I do?
    C. What does the client want from me and what sort of feeling is she or he trying to arouse in me to get it?

2. What was different within the client? Different kinds of listening to pick up whatever is live and poignant for the client at a particular moment. The emphasis is on aspects of covert experience, rather than explicit content. You can learn to listen for/observe and reflect back when appropriate:
    A. Changes in voice quality might indicate an inner focus on something that is being seen or felt differently.
    B. Highly sensory/idiosyncratic words or phrases.
    C. Aspects of content you don't actually understand and perhaps the client doesn't either.
    D. Encoded statements about other people or situations may at some level be about the client with reformulations, e.g., the client says, *"It upset me to see the little dog was alone"*. A reformulation might be, *"Seeing the little dog gave you a sense of desolation and rejection.*

Something about loneliness worries you". Reformulation to focus on the client can be practiced almost as a game in supervision.

E. Indirect or disguised communication. Anything said about something 'out there' may be about you and the helping relationship. Use immediacy (what is happening to you and me 'here-and-now').

F. Non-verbal communication, e.g., silence, gazing into space, posture. Try a hunch about the client's inner experience.

Thanks to Ian Horton for permission to reproduce the above from: Bayne, R. & Nicolson, P. (1993). *Counselling and Psychology for Health Professionals* (pp. 28–31). London: Chapman and Hall.

Appendix 7: Preparing for Supervision Using the Extended '7 Eyed' Diagram

Suggested headline for each focus:

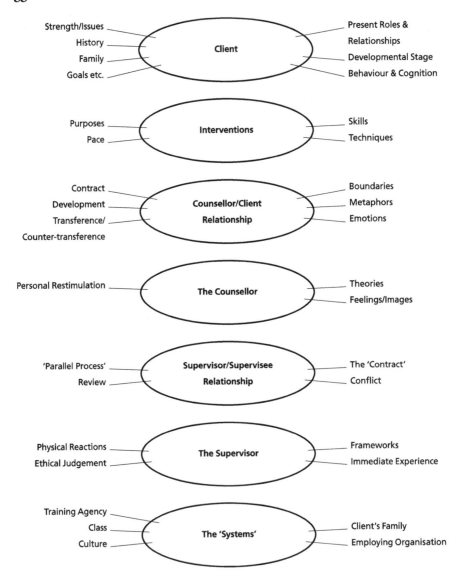

Figure 23: The Extended '7 Eyed' Diagram

Thanks to Francesca Inskipp and Brigid Proctor for permission to reproduce this from 'The Art, Craft and Tasks of Counselling Supervision', Part 2, *Becoming a Supervisor, Second Edition*, 2001, p. 62. Originally in Hawkins & Shohet (1989).

Appendix 8: Learning Styles

Descriptions of the Four Styles.

Activists

Activists like to take direct action. They are enthusiastic and welcome new challenges and experiences. They are interested primarily in the 'here-and-now'. They are less interested in what has happened in the past or in putting things into a broader context. They like to have a go, try things out and participate. They like to be the center of attention. In summary, Activists like:

1. To think on their feet.
2. To have short sessions.
3. Plenty of variety.
4. The opportunity to initiate.
5. To participate and have fun.

Reflectors

Reflectors like to think about things in detail before taking action. They take a thoughtful approach. They are good listeners and prefer to adopt a low profile. They are prepared to read and re-read and will welcome the opportunity to repeat a piece of learning. In summary, Reflectors like:

1. To think before acting.
2. Thorough preparation.
3. To research and evaluate.
4. To make decisions in their own time.
5. To listen and observe.

Theorists

Theorists like to see how things fit into an overall pattern. They are logical and objective systems people who prefer a sequential approach to problems. They are analytical, pay great attention to detail and tend to be perfectionists. In summary, Theorists like:

1. Concepts and models.
2. To see the overall picture.
3. To feel intellectually stretched.

4. Structure and clear objectives.

5. Logical presentation of ideas.

Pragmatists

Pragmatists like to see how things work in practice. They enjoy experimenting with new ideas. They are practical, down-to-earth and like to solve problems. They appreciate the opportunity to try out what they have learned/are learning. In summary, Pragmatists like:

1. To see the relevance to their work.

2. To gain practical advantage from learning.

3. Credible role models.

4. Proven techniques.

5. Activities to be real.

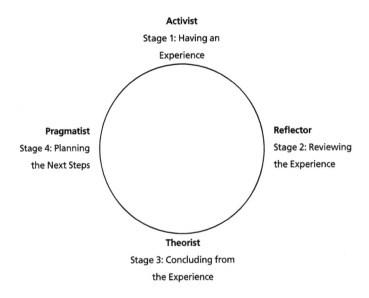

Figure 24: The Learning Styles Diagram

Thanks to Peter Honey Publications for permission to include the above descriptions of the Learning Styles. Access to the *Learning Styles Inventory* can be found at www.peterhoney.com.

Appendix 9: Questionnaire on Multiple Intelligences

Please complete the following questionnaire by assigning a numerical value to each of the statements that you consider represent you. If you agree that the statement very strongly represents you, assign a 5. If the statement does not represent you, assign a 0. Use the numbers 5–0 to grade each statement.

1. I am skilful in working with objects _____
2. I have a good sense of direction _____
3. I have a natural ability to sort out arguments between friends _____
4. I can remember the words to music easily _____
5. I am able to explain difficult topics and make them clear _____
6. I always do things one step at a time _____
7. I understand myself well and understand why I behave as I do _____
8. I enjoy community activities and social events _____
9. I learn well from talks, lectures and listening to others _____
10. When listening to music I experience changes in mood _____
11. I enjoy puzzles, crosswords, logical problems _____
12. Charts, diagrams, visual displays are important for my learning _____
13. I am sensitive to the moods and feelings of those around me _____
14. I learn best when I have to get up and do it for myself _____
15. I need to see something in front of me before I want to learn something _____
16. I like privacy and quiet for working and thinking _____
17. I can pick out individual instruments in complex musical pieces _____
18. I can visualise remembered and constructed scenes easily _____
19. I have a well-developed vocabulary and am expressive with it _____
20. I enjoy and value taking written notes _____
21. I have a good sense of balance and enjoy physical movement _____
22. I can discern pattern and relationships between experiences or things _____
23. In teams, I co-operate and build on the ideas of others _____
24. I am observant and will often see things others miss _____
25. I get restless easily _____
26. I enjoy working or learning independently of others _____

27. I enjoy making music _____
28. I have a facility with numbers and mathematical problems _____

Scoring

Enter your score for each statement, including a total for each Intelligence.

Linguistic

5 _____ 9 _____ 19 _____ 20 _____ Total _____

Mathematical and Logical

6 _____ 11 _____ 22 _____ 28 _____ Total _____

Visual and Spatial

2 _____ 12 _____ 18 _____ 24 _____ Total _____

Musical

4 _____ 10 _____ 17 _____ 27 _____ Total _____

Interpersonal

3 _____ 8 _____ 13 _____ 23 _____ Total _____

Intrapersonal

7 _____ 15 _____ 16 _____ 26 _____ Total _____

Kinesthetic

1 _____ 14 _____ 21 _____ 25 _____ Total _____

By taking the total score of each intelligence from the questionnaire, plotting it on the wheel and shading each segment you will get a visual representation of your balance of intelligences according to Howard Gardner's theory. See Gardner, H. (1999). *Intelligence reframed: Multiple intelligences for the 21st century.* New York, NY: Basic Books.

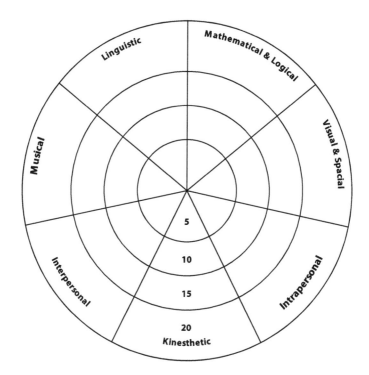

Figure 25: Multiple Intelligence Wheel

Thanks to Network Educational Press Ltd. for permission to reproduce the above questionnaire from Smith, A. (1998). *Accelerated Learning in Practice* (pp. 187–189).

Appendix 10: The Emotional Competence Framework

Personal competence (How we manage ourselves)

1. Self-awareness: Knowing one's internal states, preferences, resources and intuitions
   A. Emotional awareness: recognising one's emotions and their effects.
   B. Accurate self-assessment: knowing one's strengths and limits.
   C. Self-confidence: strong sense of one's self-worth and capabilities.

2. Self-regulation: Managing one's internal states, impulses and resources
   A. Self-control: keeping disruptive emotions and impulses in check.
   B. Trustworthiness: maintaining standards of integrity and honesty.
   C. Conscientiousness: taking responsibility for personal performance.
   D. Adaptability: flexibility in handling change.
   E. Innovation: being comfortable with novel ideas, approaches and new information.

3. Motivation: Emotional tendencies that guide or facilitate reaching goals
   A. Achievement drive: striving to improve or meet a standard of excellence.
   B. Commitment: aligning with the goals of the group or organisation.
   C. Initiative: readiness to act on opportunities.
   D. Optimism: persistence in pursuing goals despite obstacles and setbacks.

Social competence (These competencies determine how we handle relationships)

1. Empathy: Awareness of the feelings and perspectives of others and taking an active interest in their concerns
   A. Understanding others: sensing the feelings and perspectives of others, and taking an active interest in their concerns.
   B. Developing others: sensing the developmental needs of others and bolstering their abilities.
   C. Service orientation: anticipating, recognising, and meeting the needs of customers.
   D. Leveraging diversity: cultivating opportunities through different kinds of people.
   E. Political awareness: reading a group's emotional currents and power relationships.

2. Social skills: Adeptness at inducing desirable responses in others
   A. Influence: wielding effective tactics for persuasion.

B. Communication: listening openly and sending convincing messages.
C. Conflict management: negotiating and resolving disagreements.
D. Leadership: inspiring and guiding individuals and groups.
E. Change catalyst: initiating or managing change.
F. Building bonds: nurturing instrumental relationships.
G. Collaboration and cooperation: working with others toward shared goals.
H. Team capabilities: creating group synergy in pursuing collective goals.

See Goleman, D. (1998). *Working with Emotional Intelligence.* London: Bloomsbury Publishing.

Appendix 11: Feeling Words

A list of feeling words

Accepted	Afraid	Agitated	Ambivalent
Angry	Annoyed	Anxious	Arrogant
At Peace	Belittled	Blasé	Bored
Brave	Cautious	Co-Operative	Competent
Confident	Confused	Congenial	Content
Defensive	Delighted	Depressed	Disappointed
Disillusioned	Distrusting	Doubtful	Elated
Empathy	Energetic	Enthusiastic	Excited
Free	Frightened	Frustrated	Fulfilled
Genuine	Happy	Honest	Honoured
Hopeful/Less	Hurt	Ignored	Impressed
Indignant	Inferior	Inhibited	Insecure
Intolerant	Jealous	Jubilant	Jumpy
Knowledgeable	Listless	Lonely	Loving
Malevolent	Mischievous	Miserable	Moody
Morose	Nasty	Naughty	Numbed
Optimistic	Overjoyed	Overlooked	Perplexed
Picked On	Pleased	Put On	Rejected
Relaxed	Relieved	Repulsed	Resentful
Respectful	Sad	Satisfied	Shame
Shocked	Sorrow	Spiteful	Strong
Successful	Superior	Suspicious	Tense
Tolerant	Tough	Tranquil	Trusting
Unhappy	Unloved	Useful	Vain
Valiant	Valued	Vengeful	Wan
Warmth	Wary	Whimsical	Worried
Worthless	Yearning		

Please add other feeling words…

Appendix 12: Interventions to Facilitate Learning

A list of interventions to facilitate learning

Advising

Coaching

Sharing own experience

SWOT Analysis (strengths, weaknesses, opportunities, threats)

Lecturing

Interpersonal Process Recall Feedback

Drama therapy

Challenge/confront

Sculpt (animals)

Images (imaging)

Stakeholder perspectives

Circular questioning

Intuition

Play

Immediacy

Empty chair work

Socratic questioning

Suspend

Metaphor

Film

Silence (be still)

Reflection

Poetry

Instructing

Modelling

Information giving

Force-field analysis

Skills training

Role-play

Demonstrating

Draw (art)

Experiment (try differently)

Fly on wall client

Process issues

Summarising

Parallel process

Paradox

Brainstorm

Give reading

Facilitate internal reflection

Paradoxical injunctions

Narrative (Story-Telling)

Dreamwork

Scenario Planning (time paths)

Song (music)

Role-reversal

Please add other methods that would facilitate learning...

Appendix 13: Theory of Core Qualities (Ofman, 2001)

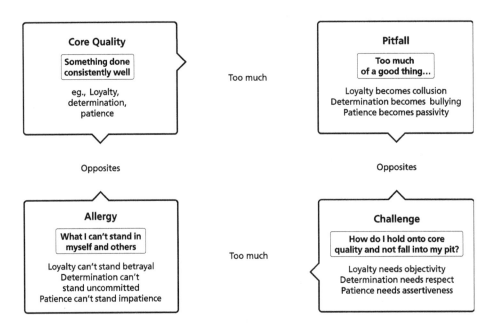

Figure 26: Theory of Core Qualities (Ofman, 2001)

My Core Quality	My Pitfall	My Challenge	My Allergy

Figure 27: Assessing my Challenges

How can I meet the challenge of holding my core quality without it falling into being too much of a good or bad thing?

Appendix 14: Drivers Checklist

Put a tick against any item that applies to you in general. Colleagues who know you well can also be invited to assist you in this process.

Please others:

1. I smile or laugh a lot when I am talking to someone □
2. I leave when things begin to go wrong to avoid conflict □
3. I nod my head a lot when I talk or frequently say "You know" □
4. I dress carefully to show that I have my own special style □
5. I laugh to smooth things over when I am a little nervous □
6. I say complimentary things before asking for something I want □
7. I act 'cheerful' to cover over my bad feelings in meetings □
8. I automatically give first priority to others whatever the situation □
9. I am usually restless when I am by myself □
10. I often volunteer to do things others are reluctant to do □

Be perfect:

1. I am very aware of the mistakes of others and often point these out □
2. I am often early for meetings and get impatient with latecomers □
3. I tidy up regularly and hesitate to use a clean waste basket □
4. I believe that attention to detail is vital to success at work □
5. I set very high standards for myself and others □
6. I collect interesting information and display this to others □
7. I get things exactly right and do not make mistakes □
8. I do not trust others to do things well enough □
9. I have difficulty in delegating tasks to others □
10. My motto is: 'If a thing is worth doing it's worth doing well' □

Be strong:

1. I am outwardly calm even when upset □
2. I consider carefully and take my time before making a decision □
3. I often do without things that I could afford or access easily □
4. I regularly carry around more in my briefcase than I need □
5. I make the best of a bad situation for far too long □
6. I do things for others that they should do for themselves □

7. I am extra cautious in most situations ☐
8. I can hide my feelings by my facial expression ☐
9. I can be physically uncomfortable for a long time without noticing too much ☐
10. I believe in not complaining in the face of adversity ☐

Hurry up:

1. I hurry even when it does not matter ☐
2. I do not get around to buying clothes that I need for work ☐
3. I am the first to say: *"Are you ready? Let's go"* ☐
4. I am quick to be on the go whatever the occasion ☐
5. I frequently tap my fingers, wiggle my feet or jiggle my knees up and down ☐
6. I do too much too fast and get exhausted ☐
7. I bump into things or people when I am in a hurry ☐
8. I interrupt people to hurry them along or start leaving before they finish ☐
9. I pace back and forth while I am waiting ☐
10. I walk fast, work fast, eat fast, and talk fast ☐

Try Hard:

1. I have trouble finishing things ☐
2. I often realise that I have done something the hard way ☐
3. I tell myself *"This time I will do it right"* and then I don't ☐
4. I have difficulty accepting when things go smoothly for others ☐
5. I delay getting around to important things for too long and sabotage myself ☐
6. I ease off the effort and delay when I get close to finishing something ☐
7. I am often disorganised and have papers strewn all over my desk ☐
8. I let jobs accumulate and then avoid them ☐
9. I am sometimes quite late for meetings or do not get there at all ☐
10. I delay too long before starting on a job ☐

Scoring

Score one point for each item that you have ticked. Scores over five will give you an indication of your 'favourite' drivers. These are the drivers that are most important to you; you can then evaluate with your coach to what extent they help or hinder your performance.

(Modelled on *'Drivers Checklist'* by Joseph William Hazell. See Hazell, J. W. (1989). Drivers as mediators of stress response. *Transactional Analysis Journal, 19*(4), 212–223.)

Appendix 15: My Learning Log

The experience:

_____

_____

_____

_____

What happened?

_____

_____

_____

What did I learn?

_____

_____

_____

How and when will I use what I have learned?

_____

_____

_____

How can I develop myself in this area?

_____

_____

_____

_____

Appendix 16: Questions to Help You Prepare for Your Supervision Session

Contracting: Starting with the end in mind and agreeing on how you will get there together

1. How do you want to use your time?
2. What do you most need to achieve in this session?
3. How could your supervisor be most valuable to you?
4. What in particular do you want to focus on during your supervision session?
5. What would make this session a success, both for you and for your organisation?
6. What do you want to have achieved or shifted before leaving here?

Generating insights into the situation

1. Are there other people involved that you have not mentioned?
2. How do other people (your client, your boss, your colleagues, your team) see the situation?
3. Can you summarise this issue?

Exploring 1: Understanding the personal impact the situation is having on you

1. How are you feeling right now?
2. Are there any feelings you have not expressed?
3. Does this person remind you of anyone?
4. What is it you would like to say to this person?
5. What in you is standing in the way of resolving this?

Exploring 2: Challenging to create new possibilities for future action in resolving the situation

1. Who might be of help to you that you have not consulted?
2. Who has the information you need?
3. Who has the skills you need?
4. Who has the power to affect change in this situation?
5. Can you think of four different ways to tackle this situation?
6. What is the wildest option you can think of to deal with this situation?
7. How would someone you admire deal with this situation?

Supporting you in committing to a way ahead and creating the next step

1. What are the pros and cons of each possible strategy?
2. What is your long-term objective?
3. What is the first step you need to take?
4. When precisely are you going to do that?
5. Who needs to be involved, consulted or informed?
6. Is your plan realistic? What is the percentage chance of you succeeding?
7. What do you need to do right now to radically increase the percentage chance of success?
8. Rehearse your opening line right now, as if I am the person you need to talk to.

Review: Taking stock

1. What have you decided to do next?
2. What have you learned from this session?
3. In what way have you increased your ability to handle similar situations?
4. What did you find helpful about this supervision process?
5. What did you find difficult about this supervision process?
6. What would you like to improve or do differently the next time you have supervision with your supervisor?
7. When are where are you going to review this experimental plan you have just committed to?
8. Are you going to have another supervision session, if so when and where?

(Adapted from Hawkins, P., & Smith, N. (2006). *Coaching, mentoring and organisational consultancy: Supervision and development.* Maidenhead, UK: Open University Press.)

Appendix 17: Supervisee Data Form

Name:

Address:

Business (address, if appropriate):

Phone numbers:

Fax numbers:

Email address:

Where best to contact you/leave messages?

Preferred means of communication:

Occupation/Job (explain a bit):

Preferred supervision schedule (telephone, face to face, etc.):

What do you want from supervision? Do you have specific goals?

What do you want to focus on first?

_____

_____

_____

How do you learn best?

_____

_____

_____

How can I facilitate your learning?

_____

_____

_____

How would I block your learning?

_____

_____

_____

Any other information that would help me in supervising you?

_____

_____

_____

Appendix 18: Reflection-in-action: Questions for the Practitioner

Questions related to problem formulation and integrative framework:

1. How would you formulate the problem that your client is presenting based in your own perspective?

2. What was your goal in this session?

3. How does this goal relate to your overall work with this person; the context of the work?

4. How would you assess your client's presentation of themselves?

5. How has this 'assessment' influenced the way in which you have approached your work with this particular person or group?

6. What was your view of the possible changes that your client may have considered?

7. Do you consider you have reached your objective in this session/in the work with this client?

8. If you work in an open-ended contract rather than a time-limited contract does this alter the way you conceptualise the work? Or vice versa?

9. In terms of the client's personality style/structure, how do you think of your work with this particular person?

10. What conversation were you having with yourself before this session? At the close of the session? How did you integrate this for yourself into an ongoing narrative?

11. Were you aware during the session of any 'enactments' on your part, or on that of the client, that may give some insight into the shared unconscious process between you and your client?

12. What are the values that inform your view of your work and, in particular, of the process of change?

13. Discuss how an awareness of issues of difference informed your process in this piece of work?

14. What in particular do you consider that you bring to the work with this client?

15. How do you take into account the contextual factors that impact on your work with this client?

16. What might be the cost of 'change' to the client/to the client's family?

17. When may 'enactments' become an ethical issue?

Questions related to particular interventions:

1. Did your intervention achieve the desired outcome?
2. If so, how did this further your work with the client? How do you assess whether your intervention is effective? What criteria do you use?
3. How do you judge whether an intervention has been ineffective or 'missed' your client?
4. What do you keep in mind when considering the next intervention?
5. Choose an intervention that you consider effective and give reasons for your choice.
6. Focus on an intervention where you 'missed' your client and there was a 'rupture' in your alliance. Consider the implications of this event, alternative responses and the possible unconscious enactment in this process. How will you address this process of 'rupture and repair'?

Checklist for counter transference responses to the client:

1. What am I feeling in response to the client?
2. Do these feelings confirm or conflict with other impressions I have of this client?
3. On balance, do these feelings tell me more about the client or about myself?
4. Do I want to feed these feelings back to the client?
5. What is making me want to feed back? Or not, as the case may be?
6. Would feedback, in my opinion, benefit or hurt the client?
7. Is this the most appropriate time to talk this through?
8. Should the feelings be fed back in the form of interpretations?
9. Should I disclose my feelings directly through self-disclosure or simply interpret what the client may fear that I am feeling?

Reflection-in-action: Consider the following stages of the process of reflection in your thinking about this therapeutic work (Schon, 1983)

1. What are the unique features of this client's situation? How do you understand the problem that is facing you and your client? What values concerning change inform your problem formulation? What is your initial tentative 'story' regarding the journey the two of you will embark upon? How have you arrived at this 'story'?

2. From your own past experience—work with clients; reading case studies in books and journals; your personal work, self-awareness and experience— you have built up a repertoire of understandings, images, metaphors, examples, stories and actions that may be relevant in some way to this client. What familiar situation/picture may serve as an exemplar for this unfamiliar situation? Carefully consider the similarities and differences.

3. What exploratory 'experiment' emerges from these reflections that may facilitate an agreed change? What 'discovery' arises from your interaction? What do you learn from the client's responses?

4. How do you integrate the outcome of your intervention, this new discovery, into your ongoing reflective process so that you remain open to the ever-changing, interactive nature of the emergent story? Are you tempted to adhere to your hypothesis in the face of contradictory 'evidence'? If so, what are your reflections in this instance on your own counter transference?

5. Are you aware of the way in which the process between you and the client may reflect aspects of the client's experience in the 'world out there'? (And how this may be true for you too?)

Compiled by Maria Gilbert, September 2006.

(Any further suggestions will be welcome).

Appendix 19: The Six Levels of Reflection

Level 1

Zero reflection/me-stance/disconnection

Level 1 is a non-reflective stance—*"I am right, you are way off the mark"*. This level of reflection finds it difficult to go internal, or to look at wider pictures or bigger systems. It has a black-and-white stance to making sense of events and is based on a theory of causality that is very simple, such as 'this caused that to happen'. There is no awareness of circular causality here, of where cause and effect intertwine. The answer we seek usually is straightforward: *"If you would change, my life would be easier"*.

"I'm OK (could be I'm not OK), you're not OK." A position of blame is often adopted. This easily can be a victim stance: *"See how badly the world treats me!"* We call this the 'me-stance (external)' because it focuses on the actor/person, but from an external perspective. There is little consideration for how I might be part of the problem or contribute to it. *"By and large at this stage—you are the problem, I am the solution."*

Level 2

Empathic reflection/observer stance/empathic connection

Level 2 reflection sees the reflector becoming more of an observer with acknowledgement of feelings. There is a movement from event to personality. There is an awareness of some empathy for the other person's perspective or for another perspective. A more compassionate interpretation allows for insights into what is happening to the other.

"I'm OK (could still be I'm not OK) and realising you might be OK (but not yet). You are still the problem and I am still, by and large the solution." A position of blame plus understanding (some empathy) is most common.

Level 3

Relational reflection/you-and-me = us stance/personal connection

Level 3 often follows a dialogue (internal or external) where we begin to share the issues and see that many of the issues or problems are relational. *"Now I see that it's about you and me and how we are getting on together."* Or we begin to see that the issue or the problem we are facing is, in fact, relational rather than simply part of one person. While we both bring our personal histories into this shared space, there is an awareness that we create a relational dilemma for which we both have some responsibility. *"We can work out a way of working together."*

"We are OK if we can talk about it." Position is one of collective responsibility. An 'us' stance. *"We have a problem and we have the solution."*

Level 4

Systemic reflection/you-and-me + others/contextual connection

This is the systemic reflective stance that looks to the system, and the various subsystems involved. It allows us to reflect on the situation from these perspectives. It is the helicopter (or satellite) ability to see the various small and large systems that affect our lives and our behaviours. Level 4 reflection looks for the connections between the 'you' and the 'me' that create the larger 'us'. This extends beyond our immediate dyad, team or group to the shared resources and history that shape/influence our choices and values. Level 4 can extend our reflective inquiry into ancestry, heritage, community, culture and ecosystem.

"We're OK." Position is one of systemic responsibility. The bigger picture stance. How is it all connected and how can we see and reflect from these multiple perspectives?

Level 5

Self-reflection/me (internalised) stance/incorporating connection

This self-transcendent position means I begin to look at me and consider how I set up these situations. *"Gosh!, it's actually about me!"* This position looks at how insight, and my awareness of myself, results in ways of working that involve changing my mind set, and my meaning-making perspectives. I can change, and if I change, then we all have the opportunity to experience ourselves and the situation differently. Thinking intersubjectively (relationality), but in a way that helps me see my part in this.

"I'm OK, you're OK." Position is one of personal responsibility. The me-stance (internal). *"I have issues and problems I need to resolve."* Unlike Level 1, which is also a 'me' position but external to me, Level 5 goes internal to articulate my own patterns and themes that contribute to the way I engage in life and relationships.

Level 6

Transcendent reflection/other (universal stance)/universal connection

This is the reflective stance that sees 'beyond' to what makes meaning and what gives meaning to life. It transcends any particular relationship, person or situation, opening into a larger construct that is inherent in all relationships, people, or situations. For many, this can be a religious or spiritual stance that reflects a philosophy or a system of meaning that already exists (e.g, Christianity, Judaism), or one that I create (my philosophy of life). It can be seen as what gives meaning to life, people and behaviour, e.g., that God loves us, that suffering exists, that individuals have value in themselves. It adopts an existential position on life often called the '*Transpersonal*' or '*Transcendent*'. It can be theistically-based or not.

There is a higher or larger perspective that helps me make sense of life and purpose (e.g., humanistic, atheistic, denominational religion, Buddhist). I find meaning by subscribing to this existential position. I attempt to live the current situation through this expanded perspective, and recognise my own personal limitations of perception. I have a clear intention to expand my 'little self' and embody more of the qualities of transcendence that guide, teach and inspire me. I am willing to adopt this expanded view/state of being, even though it may require me to enter a space of 'not knowing', and may engender a profound restructuring of my mental constructs.

Appendix 20: Incisive Questions (Nancy Kline & Others, 1999)

You assume you are stupid: If you knew you were intelligent how would you talk to...

1. If you knew you could do that, what thoughts would you have?
2. If you knew you could do that, what would change, what new ideas would you have, how would you feel?
3. What more/else do you think, feel or say?
4. What might we be assuming here that limits our thinking? On this issue?
5. What might you have noticed that needs attention or change in this company that I may have missed? What do you think should be done about it?
6. If you were the CEO what problem would you solve first and how would you do it?
7. If you knew what was essential to your company's success, how would you approach your work?
8. If things were to be right for you at work, what would need to change?
9. If you were to not hold back at work (in your team) what would change for you?
10. If you could say what you really wanted to say, what would it be?
11. If you knew you were respected, what would you do or say?
12. What do you think you have accomplished in this period?
13. What in particular has gone well?
14. What are you proud of?
15. What have you discovered about yourself?
16. What is the key thing you want to improve?
17. What are you assuming could stop you doing what you want to do?
18. What support do you need from me to do that?
19. What do you think your next learning goals should be?
20. What other issues do you want to raise with me?
21. If it were up to you what changes would you like to see in our relationship?
22. What do you really think?
23. If you were in my position, what would you do that I am not doing?

24. What assumptions are we making that limit everything?

25. What would you like to achieve here? Now? Later?

26. What would you like to be remembered for?

27. What are we not facing that is right in front of us?

28. How would your work have to change to be right for you?

29. What do I assume about myself that is limiting me?

30. If I weren't afraid, what would I be risking?

31. If I were to be really *me* here, what would I be doing differently?

32. What are you assuming that allows you to ignore this?

33. If you were to face it, what positive outcomes might result?

34. If you knew that you could handle the fallout, what steps would you take to live free of this denial?

Appendix 21: Statement of Best Ethical Practice

The UK branch of the *International Coach Federation*, the *Association for Professional Executive Coaching and Supervision*, the *European Mentoring and Coaching Council UK*, and the *Association for Coaching* (AC), signed a statement *'synthesising the best ethical practice of all the professional bodies'* at a meeting on 28 January, 2008.

Statement of shared professional values

Purpose

This statement has been agreed by the coaching professional bodies in the UK who cooperate to enhance the reputation of the coaching industry.

In the emerging profession of coaching, we believe that:

1. Every coach, whether charging fees for coaching provided to individuals or organisations or both, is best served by being a member of a professional body suiting his/her needs.

2. Every coach needs to abide by a code of governing ethics and apply acknowledged standards to the performance of their coaching work.

3. Every coach needs to invest in their ongoing continuing professional development to ensure the quality of their service and their level of skill is enhanced.

4. Every coach has a duty of care to ensure the good reputation of our emerging profession.

The following are fundamental principles by which we expect our members to operate:

5. **Meta Principle** To continually enhance the competence and reputation of the coaching profession.

6. **Principle One: Reputation** Every coach will act positively and in a manner that increases the public's understanding and acceptance of coaching

7. **Principle Two: Continuous competence enhancement** Every coach accepts the need to enhance their experience, knowledge, capability and competence on a continuous basis

8. **Principle Three: Client centred** Every client is creative, resourceful and whole, and the role of the coach is to keep the development of that

client central to his/her work, and ensure that all services provided are appropriate to the needs of the client.

9. **Principle Four: Confidentiality and standards** Every coach has a professional responsibility (beyond the terms of the contract with the client) to apply high standards in their service provision and behaviour. He/she needs to be open and frank about methods and techniques used in the coaching process, maintain only appropriate records and to respect the confidentiality; a) of the work with their clients; and b) or their representative body's members information.

10. **Principle Five: Law and diversity** Every coach will act within the Laws of the jurisdictions within which they practice and will also acknowledge and promote diversity at all times.

11. **Principle Six: Boundary management** Every coach will recognise their own limitations of competence and the need to exercise boundary management. The rights of the client to terminate the coaching process will be respected at all times, as will the need to acknowledge different approaches to coaching which may be more effective for the client than their own. Every endeavour will be taken to ensure the avoidance of conflicts of interest.

12. **Principle Seven: Personal pledge** Every coach will undertake to abide by the above principles that will complement the principles, codes of ethics and conduct set out by their own representative body to which they adhere and by the breach of which they would be required to undergo due process.

Published 25 February, 2008.

About the Authors

Michael Carroll Ph.D.

Michael is a Fellow of the British Association for Counselling, a Chartered Counselling Psychologist and a BACP Senior Registered Practitioner. He is an Accredited Executive Coach and an Accredited Executive Coach Supervisor with APECS (Association for Professional Executive Coaches and Supervisors). Michael is Visiting Industrial Professor in the Graduate School of Education, University of Bristol and the winner of the 2001 British Psychological Society Award for Distinguished Contributions to Professional Psychology. He is author or co-author of: *'Training Counselling Supervisors: Strategies, Methods, Techniques'*; *'Counselling Supervision in Context'*; *'The Handbook of Counselling in Organisations'*; *'Counselling Supervision: Theory, Skills and Practice'*; *'Workplace Counselling'*; *'Integrative Approaches to Supervision'*; *'Becoming an Executive Coachee: Creating Learning Partnerships'*; and *'On Being a Supervisee: Creating Learning Partnerships'*.

Email: MCarr1949@aol.com

Maria Gilbert M.A.

Maria C. Gilbert is a UKCP registered Integrative Psychotherapist, a Chartered Psychologist (BPS), a Registered Clinical Psychologist (HPC), an APECS Accredited Executive Coach, an Accredited Member of the Society for Coaching Psychology, a BACP Senior Accredited Supervisor and a visiting Professor at Middlesex University, who is currently joint head of the Integrative Department with Vanja Orlans, and a programme leader with Simon Cavicchia on the MA/MSc in Coaching Psychology, at Metanoia Institute. Over the years she has co-authored several books: *'Brief Therapy with Couples'*; *'Psychotherapy Supervision'*; *'An Introduction to Integrative Psychotherapy'*; *'On Becoming a Supervisee: Creating Learning Partnerships'*; *'Becoming an Executive Coachee: Creating Learning Partnerships'*; and most recently, *'Integrative Therapy: 100 Key Points and Techniques'*.

Email: maria@fluffy.dircon.co.uk

CPSIA information can be obtained
at www.ICGtesting.com
Printed in the USA
LVHW052026100623
749439LV00003B/75